# BOOMERWALK™

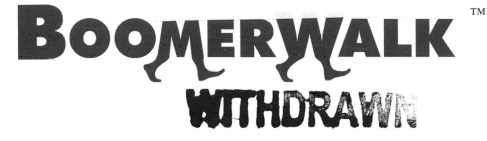

## Why Baby Boomers Should Replace Running and Jogging with Racewalking

D0573358

## Brent Bohlen

**Walking Promotions**
**Medford, NJ**

Cover Photo: The cover photo and all photographs of Max Walker and Cathy Mayfield illustrating racewalking technique were taken by Michael K. Smeltzer. Photos of profiled racewalkers were provided by the subjects. Some additional photos are credited individually.

Printed in the USA
First Edition

# Dedication

To Mary, the woman I married at age 20 and happily would marry again nearly four decades later. Every man should be so fortunate.

# Foreword

When Brent Bohlen first contacted me with the concept of *BoomerWalk,* it quickly became obvious that this racewalking book was completely different from the current crop of racewalking texts. Instead of focusing on the minutia of racewalking technique, *BoomerWalk* is an inspiring look at the author's discovery of racewalking as one of more than 70 million baby boomers.

While everyone is aware of the benefits of regular exercise, many baby boomers do not heed the sage advice to get the heart pumping regularly. Some exercised before, but their bodies have broken down. Some walk, but do not get their hearts pumping hard enough. Still others have never exercised. Regardless of which group you fall into, *BoomerWalk* motivates you to get moving, really moving. Bohlen's racewalking uses 95% of your muscles and easily gets your heart rate into the required target zone to maximize aerobic benefits without undue stress on your joints, ligaments, and tendons.

Bohlen's BoomerWalk portrays his awakening to the benefits of racewalking as well as shares encouraging stories of other racewalkers who range in age from their 50s to their 90s. His explanation of racewalking along with large photographs combine to effectively illustrate how to racewalk as well as describe the supporting exercises that get you off the couch and fit for the rest of your life. Make Bohlen's vision of a healthy, energetic baby boomer population come to fruition. Read this book and, more importantly, go out and walk.

Jeff Salvage, Founder **www.racewalk.com**

# Acknowledgments

I entered my first racewalking event without any knowledge of the sport and received my first instruction on the rules at the starting line. I talked with fellow racewalkers after the competition. During the next year couple of years I visited racewalking Web sites, read and watched racewalking expert Jeff Salvage's *Race Walk Like a Champion* book and DVD, took one of Dave McGovern's "World Class" racewalking clinics, experienced an impromptu session with legendary coach Frank Alongi and continued conversations with racewalkers I met.

Nearly all of what I know about racewalking I learned from others. While I identify some people in the text as the source of specific racewalking concepts, it would be impossible for me to attribute many of the insights that came from dozens of casual conversations during the past few years. The remainder of my knowledge is based on experience – the legacy of mistakes I made and, no doubt, will continue to make.

I am indebted to many individuals who provided information for the racewalker profiles sandwiched between chapters. More volunteered their experiences with the sport than I had room to include. Their willingness to contribute is typical of racewalkers' benevolent sharing of knowledge with fellow enthusiasts. If you are interested in reading more profiles or sending us your story, please visit www.boomerwalk.com.

Max Walker and Cathy Mayfield, who each set national age-group records in the 50K racewalk, generously agreed to be photographed to illustrate racewalking technique. When I started I could hold form no more than 400 meters (1/4 of a mile). These baby boomer athletes walk with speed and grace for 31 miles. Longtime friend and photojournalist Mike Smeltzer contributed his expertise in capturing the essential points of racewalking. Matt Stolze, a talented, young graphic artist, developed the footed BoomerWalk logo. Whatever writing skills I have are primarily because of many years of help from my journalist/professor wife, Mary.

I owe special thanks to and have great admiration for Jeff Salvage and Dave McGovern. I contacted these world-class racewalkers, coaches and authors of their own excellent books on racewalking to explain my intentions with the book and to see if they would be interested in reviewing the manuscript. Both immediately agreed. I am honored these authorities took the time to examine the draft. The final product is much improved and is more useful to the reader because of their thoughtful input.

Finally, Jeff Salvage and his publishing arm, Walking Promotions, were instrumental to bringing this book to print. Jeff's keen understanding of the process, sharp focus on the task, vast knowledge of the subject matter and sympathetic touch with the author made the publishing experience a joy.

# Contents

# Racewalker Profiles

I inserted profiles of racewalkers between chapters. These racewalkers represent a sample that could be repeated many times, and I received more stories than I could use in the book. The youngest are in their mid-50s. Others are older than baby boomers but serve as inspirations for us. One is in her 90s and still competes in national races. We all hope to live to such an age, and we should aspire to be as vigorous as she.

I met some of these athletes at races when I was competing, and I contacted others through racewalking clubs around the country. Because of the manner in which I met them, most are avid competitors and members of clubs. Competing and being a member of a club can enhance your racewalking experience, but neither is necessary for you to enjoy the benefits of this sport. I don't have a club within 100 miles of my home, and yet I love the activity. I would continue racewalking for fitness if I never entered a race again.

Some of the racewalkers are relatively new to the sport while others have been at it for decades. They discovered the sport in various ways, and each had his or her own reason for taking up racewalking. Several received injuries from running or other sports and found racewalking a "joint-friendly" alternative. Some have experienced no injuries racewalking other than an occasional ache or pain from vigorous training or competition. Others have had mostly transient minor injuries that are surprisingly rare for the number of years and number of miles of training they have put into the sport.

A few of the racewalkers were exceptional athletes in other sports but most were not. They all are reaping the benefits of this aerobic activity, and many are doing extraordinary things. Perhaps you will recognize yourself in one or more of the profiles. For every one of these racewalkers many others are participating on a regular basis in clubs, with friends or on their own. You also can benefit from racewalking, and maybe you will soon be doing extraordinary things as well.

Racewalker profiles follow these chapters:

**Chapter One**
Jean Brunnenkant took up the sport at 75 and still wins gold medals in her 90s.
William A. Riley, Jr., a 50-something former runner with bad knees, shaped up and got a new wardrobe.

**Chapter Two**
Donese Mayfield, a musician and self-described as "not an athlete," completed a marathon and two half marathons.
Dr. Alan Poisner, now in his 70s, works out five days a week and completes two half marathons a year.

**Chapter Three**
Lynn Tracy didn't let arthritis and breast cancer prevent her from setting an American record.
Charles M. Williams began racewalking after a running injury and now tries to get older runners to switch to racewalking "before they disintegrate from injuries."

**Chapter Four**
Sandy Lawson joined a club to learn racewalking technique after being disqualified in her first race.
Ryszard Nawrocki received his racewalking instruction from a famous teacher.

# Introduction

I'm a baby boomer, and if you picked up this book, you probably are, too. The group born from 1946 to 1964 is the 800-pound gorilla of demographics. We dominate and change our culture as we move through life's stages.

The boomers' obsession with youth and fitness brought many of us to the cusp of retirement in good physical condition and in anticipation of continued active lifestyles. That's me, and there's a good chance that's you, too. (If you are out of shape, keep reading. This book also is for you.)

Unfortunately, decades of running and jumping and twisting and turning took a toll on my body, especially my knees. I gave up basketball for the final time in my early 50s. A few days of jogging left my knees weak and tender. The lateral motion of tennis was out of the question.

I was mourning losses in my life – loss of the ability to do activities that I loved, loss of vigor from not being able to stay in good aerobic condition and loss of the challenge of athletic competition. But the confluence of three events helped me find a way to fill the void left by the sports I could no longer continue:

- I discovered that I can walk a lot without my knees getting sore.
- I read the book *Younger Next Year* and realized I needed to get my heart rate up for an extended period six days a week.
- I went as a spectator to the Illinois Senior Olympics and saw a racewalking competition.

Because I already was walking at a pretty good clip on a treadmill at the local fitness club several days a week, I thought I could compete with some of the walkers I saw in the state senior Olympics. The following year I signed up for the event. Without any research or instruction in racewalking, I thought my brisk-paced walking would be enough to prepare me for the Illinois Senior Olympics. Somewhere I picked up the notion that the only rule for racewalking was that at least one foot always must be in contact with the ground. Otherwise, one is running.

When the dozen or so competitors were called to the starting line of the 1,500 meter race, a woman in an official-looking red, white and blue outfit gave instructions. "There are two rules in racewalking," she began.

Uh-oh. I had a bit of that sinking feeling in my stomach I get when I dream that I forgot to go to a college class all semester.

The second requirement, it turns out, is that your lead leg must be straightened at the knee at the time your heel strikes the ground, and your leg must remain straightened at the knee until your leg passes vertically under your body. At the time it sounded weird to me, as it probably does to you now. The official went on to say that judges stationed around the track watch for infractions of the rules, and if three judges give an athlete a "red card" for a rule violation, they will disqualify the walker.

Before I had a chance to reconsider what I had gotten myself into and step off the track, the gun went off. Two of the racewalkers took off at such a clip that I could not have kept up if I were running. I would have stopped to watch them, but I was in a race. I'm a competitor. People were behind me, and I had to stay ahead of them. I tried to straighten my lead leg on every stride, but as I approached the first curve on the track 100 meters into the race the judge flashed a yellow warning paddle at me and called out "Bent knee."

Dang. I tried harder to make sure my knee was straightened. Another yellow paddle warning or two came my way during the race. I had seen real racewalkers on TV a few times and had tried imitating them in practice. It was exhausting, and I knew I could only walk fast in that style for one lap of the three and three-quarter lap race. When I got to the last lap I started my imitation of a real racewalker.

I came in third overall with a time of 10 minutes and 10.8 seconds. I didn't know it at the time, but the two individuals who took off so fast, David Couts of Missouri and Dr. Robert Shires of Iowa, are national-caliber racewalkers. They beat me by more than two minutes and showed me that racewalking can be a competitive sport performed by superior athletes.

I found out after the race that I didn't get any red cards. The judge who gave the pre-race instructions said I should have walked the entire race the way I did the last lap. I had to confess that I physically couldn't have walked the whole distance that way. That St. Louis-based official USA Track & Field judge, Ginger Mulanax, is a great friend of the sport and later helped me with racewalkers I was training.

Knowing I needed to learn more about race walking, upon arriving home I sought information from the Internet and practiced what I learned. I went back the Illinois Senior Olympics the next year and qualified for the following summer's biennial National Senior Games in Louisville, Kentucky.

I didn't want to be embarrassed on a national stage. Perhaps I had survived two state senior Olympics without disqualification, but would my form be sufficiently legal at a higher level? Would all of the competitors be blazingly fast like Couts and Shires?

I got Jeff Salvage's book and DVD on racewalking. His outstanding photos and video clips illustrated the finer points of technique. I knew what to do. It was up to me to implement it. I was particularly struck by his admonition to avoid imitating another particular racewalker because everyone's body is unique. Use good technique but apply it to your personal body structure and strengths.

Dave McGovern held a weekend clinic a four-hour drive away in Indianapolis so I signed up. We had instruction on the track and in the classroom. I continue to get new insights when I refer back to my

3

notes. But what most impressed me from the weekend was the incredible fluidity of one of the other participants. She flew along, yet her feet moved as smoothly as if she were peddling a bicycle.

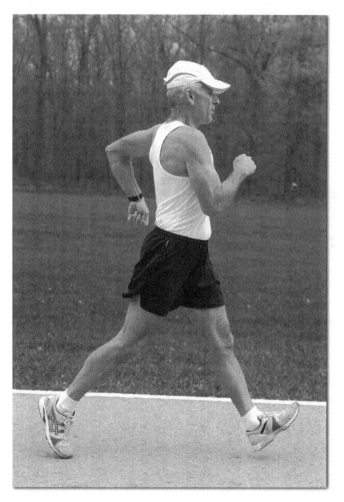

*Figure I - 1: Max Walker, shown in full stride,
exhibits proper racewalking form.*

I kept on practicing. Finally, it was time for the 2007 National Senior Games in Louisville. I knew I didn't have a chance for a top-three medal, but I hoped to place in the top eight and get a ribbon. I surprised myself, placing fifth in my age group in both the 1,500 meter and 5K races.[*] My time in the 1,500 meter racewalk was 9 minutes and 10.76 seconds, a minute faster than in my first race at the 2005 Illinois Senior Olympics. I finished the 5K in 32 minutes and 36.86 seconds. Those weren't great times, but one of the advantages of being in a sport that has yet to mushroom in popularity is that modest times can still earn ribbons. Couts and Shires, who so impressed me in my first race nearly two years earlier, won both distances in the 50-54 and 55-59 age groups, respectively.

Our generation put fitness into mainstream culture. I remember when jogging first started to gain popularity. People thought it looked odd. But no one thinks that jogging looks odd now. Admittedly, racewalking looks a bit funny at first, too. If baby boomers discover racewalking, in a few years no one will think it seems odd either. We'll be much healthier because of it, and, if we choose, we can still be competing decades from now.

Maybe you were part of the running craze and the years of pounding on the pavement have taken a toll on your body. Perhaps you used to get exercise in other sports but you've had to give them up as you've aged. Or maybe you've never been very active and you need to improve your health and lose weight. For all of you, racewalking is what you need.

---

*More than 12,000 senior athletes participated in many different sports at the National Senior Games in Louisville in 2007. The officials awarded eight places in each event. Although I'm quite proud that I placed in the two racewalking events, I have no illusion that I'm the fifth fastest racewalker in the nation between the ages of 55 and 59. Many excellent racewalkers don't come to the Games. And the 60-64 age group often has superior competition because more walkers are retired and thus have more time to train and can get away for the Games. If I had been in the 60-64 age group in 2007 with the same times, I would have finished 11th in each race.*

I need to add a special comment for men. Bonnie Stein, who taught thousands to racewalk during the past twenty years, told me women are happy to embrace racewalking once she has explained the benefits of the sport. But she finds men are stubbornly resistant to move from running to racewalking even when they suffer nagging injuries.

Here's my pitch to those men who think they are too macho for racewalking: I came from a family of athletes and learned to pole vault when I was six. By the third grade I earned a varsity letter on the junior high track team. I participated in various competitive sports for five decades. Running the quarter mile in high school was the most physically unpleasant competitive event I participated in on a regular basis and is at the top of my macho scale. But racewalking is as technically and aerobically challenging as any sport I attempted. Please don't let your preconceptions prevent you from discovering this terrific sport.

# Chapter One: Why Should Baby Boomers Racewalk?

The sport of racewalking can do for you and millions of other baby boomers what it does for me and for several thousand racewalkers young and old. You will burn calories and get wonderful cardiovascular exercise, but the joints in your body won't be abused like they are from running and jogging. If you want competition, you can find it locally and nationally.

## Highly Aerobic

Racewalking isn't just a walk in the park. It's vigorous. That's what makes it ideal as an aerobic exercise. I train at a heart rate of 125 to 150 beats per minute (BPM). When I'm in a 1,500 meter (0.93 miles) race my heart rate tops 160 BPM for about nine minutes. My heart rate is about 155 BPM for more than 30 minutes in a 5K (3.1 miles) race and approximately 145 BPM for more than an hour in a 10K (6.2 miles) race. **Because racewalking can be so intense, check with your doctor to make certain you are up to the activity before you begin racewalking.**

I'm not sure whether a rule against recommending another book in the first chapter of a book exists, but if it does, I'm going to break it. If you are a baby boomer and are concerned about living a long and healthy life, you should read *Younger Next Year*.[1] The authors provide an entertaining and convincing case for regular aerobic exercise as a key to a vigorous life well into old age. If you need a boost to get you going, this book should do it.

In *Younger Next Year* authors Crowley and Lodge recommend aerobic exercise that maintains your heart rate at 60 percent to 65 percent of your maximum heart rate for 45 minutes six days a week[2]. You can substitute vigorous weight training on two of the six days. You probably already know the widely touted benefits of weight training, including greater muscle strength, increased bone density and better coordination and balance. Dr. Lodge examines the science of enhancing neural networks through weight training and concludes, "Aerobic exercise saves your life; strength training makes it worth living.[3]"

You would not want to begin a regimen as rigorous as recommended in *Younger Next Year* without your doctor's approval. Depending on your physical condition when you begin, it may take a while to build up to the level recommended by Crowley and Lodge.

Racewalking exercises 95 percent of the muscles in the body while running uses only about 70 percent.[4] Proper racewalking technique involves substantial movement of the arms, hips, legs and feet. Try racewalking, and you'll soon discover it takes more effort from more parts of your body to racewalk at a given pace than to run or jog.

---

[1] Crowley, Chris and Lodge, Henry S., M.D., Younger Next Year: A Guide to Living Like 50 Until Your're 80 and Beyond, New York: Workman Publishing, 2004. If you are a woman, read the sequel, Younger Next Year for Women: Live Like You're 50 – Strong, Fit, Sexy – Until Your're 80 and Beyond. Note: The paperback versions both have the subtitle Live Strong, Fit, and Sexy – Until You're 80 and Beyond.

[2] Crowley and Lodge, p. 128.

[3] Crowley and Lodge, p. 178.

[4] Salvage, Jeff. *Racewalk Like a Champion*, Medford, NJ: Walking Promotions, 2004, p. 7.

The Physical Activity Guidelines for Americans issued in October 2008 by the U.S. Department of Health and Human Services recognize the aerobic benefits of racewalking:

> Adults gain substantial health benefits from two and one half hours a week of moderate intensity aerobic physical activity, or one hour and fifteen minutes of vigorous physical activity. Walking briskly, water aerobics, ballroom dancing and general gardening are examples of moderate intensity aerobic activities. Vigorous intensity aerobic activities include **racewalking**, jogging or running, swimming laps, jumping rope and hiking uphill or with a heavy backpack. (Emphasis added.)

Perhaps I tend to emphasize the cardiovascular benefits of racewalking because of my strong family history of heart disease. However, you can't have lived in our society without being aware that an aerobic, weight-bearing exercise that involves movements of many joints also can have benefits for weight control, diabetes, bone density, arthritis and many other indicators of general health.

## Low Impact

You probably know of people who gave up running because their knees or other joints couldn't take the abuse anymore. Runners' and joggers' joints endure a lot of stress step after step, mile after mile, year after year. Look at the head of a runner or jogger sometime and notice how it goes up and down with each step. That gives some idea of the pounding that is going on lower in the body.

If you watch a racewalker you'll see lots of movement in the legs, the hips, the arms and the torso, but the head remains almost perfectly still. There isn't much up and down pounding.

A racewalker keeps the advancing foot low to the ground, and the foot doesn't strike with much force. Stress on ligaments, tendons and muscles is minimized because the knee is not bent when the foot makes contact. Less impact and less stress mean less injury. According to the North American Racewalking Foundation Web site, a racewalker's heel impacts at about one and one-half times body weight while a runner's heel impact is three and one-half times body weight. [5]

"Anything that increases the forces across a joint is going to accelerate the load on the cartilage and increase the risk of osteoarthritis," said Diane Hillard-Sembell, M.D., an orthopedic surgeon, knee and sports medicine specialist and medical director of AthletiCare, a sports medicine and performance program in Springfield, Illinois. "It is estimated that knee joint loads may reach 5 to 8 times body weight during jogging and even up to 14 times body weight with fast running. Racewalking would seem to produce less forces on the knee and less potential for damage because of its straight knee and less vertical motion," she said.

Research confirms that racewalking is a relatively injury-free activity. An article in the Journal of Athletic Training[6] related a study where researchers collected information from 400 racewalkers. The subjects were 12 to 88 years old and had racewalked as little as 3 months to as long as 62 years. Nearly three-quarters were male. More than one-third began racewalking because of an injury in another sport.

On average the racewalkers in the study reported 1 injury every 6.4 years. That included minor injuries that had little effect on their racewalking activity. Only half of the injuries, or an average of about 1 every 13 years of participation, affected their training. Serious injuries in which the person had "pain all the time, eliminating all exercise and

---

[5] "Racewalking Shoes," n.d., http://www.philsport.com/narf/ashoes.htm (21 August 2008)

[6] Francis P, Richman N and Patterson P. Injuries in the Sport of Racewalking. *J Athl Train.* 1998;33(2):122-129.

affecting many daily activities" occurred on average once in 51.7 years of racewalking, according to the article.

If you've been a runner or an athlete in about any other sport, you know that is a comparatively low injury rate. That is supported by a review of the abstracts of research studies at www.pubmed.gov. A study of 4,358 male joggers found 45.8 percent had injuries during a one-year period,[7] and another study of 1,680 male and female runners showed 48 percent reported injuries in a year.[8] Those studies indicate an expected running or jogging injury about every two years, three times the rate in the racewalker study. A survey of 10 separate studies of running injuries found annual injury rates from 24 percent to 65 percent,[9] or an injury every one and one-half years to every four years – all more frequent than the injuries reported in the Richman-Patterson study of the 400 racewalkers.

Some other discoveries by the researchers in the racewalker study are enlightening. The incidence of injuries was essentially the same for men and women. Racewalkers under age 30 had higher rates of injury, as did those who walked six or seven days a week rather than three days or less. Also, the greatest number of injuries involved those who walked more than 50 miles per week, and those who walked less than 15 miles a week had the least.

While several research studies have looked at energy expended by elite racewalkers, I wish more data existed comparing racewalking and running on parameters important to average participants such as injury rates and forces applied to various parts of the body. Dr. Hillard-Sembell and her group are in the early phases of a biomechanical force plate study that should provide some comparative

---

[7] Marti B, Vader JP, Minder CE, Abelin T. On the Epidemiology of Running Injuries. The 1984 Bern Grand-Prix Study. *Am J Sports Med.* 1988 May-Jun;16(3):285-94.

[8] Walter SD, Hart LE, McIntosh JM, Sutton JR. The Ontario Cohort Study of Running-Related Injuries. *Arch Intern Med.* 1989 Nov;149(11):2561-4.

[9] Hoeberigs JH. Factors Related to the Incidence of Running Injuries. A Review. *Sports Med.* 1992 June;13(6):408-22.

data. I challenge other sports medicine researchers to initiate studies directly comparing racewalking with running and jogging.

**Please note:** In spite of the fact that racewalking is a low-impact activity compared to running and jogging, injuries can and do occur. Different people's bodies react to stresses differently. If you do get injured, address the issue by seeing a medical professional.

## Competition If You Want It

Racewalking has a long history as a competitive sport and has been an Olympic event since 1908. The current Olympic version is not for the faint of heart. Women compete in a 20K (12.4 miles) race, and men compete at 20K and 50K (31 miles). The world record time in the latter race, which is nearly 5 miles longer than a marathon, is just more than 3 hours and 34 minutes. That's 6 minutes and 55 seconds per mile for 31 miles without running!

A 50K race at the world-class level is not the type of competition that interests you and me – well, at least not me. I want competition that is fun, that provides purpose for my training and that perhaps gives me a chance at earning a ribbon or medal. The opportunities to compete are out there, and the chapter on competition will help you find them.

Dave Couts, one of the athletes who blasted away from the starting line in my first competition, made an interesting observation about runners who become racewalkers. He said there isn't necessarily a direct correlation between one's aptitude as a runner and as a racewalker. Excellent road runners may make average racewalkers, and average road runners may make exellent racewalkers. If you are an average road runner, perhaps racewalking is a sport in which you can excel.

## The Purpose of This Book

It's not my goal to turn you into an Olympic racewalk medalist. The purpose of this book is to get you and tens of thousands of other baby boomers to begin racewalking and start enjoying the benefits of this sport. If just 1 in 1,000 of the 75 million baby boomers takes it up, we'll have 75,000 new racewalkers. What if 1 in 100 started racewalking? Or 1 in 10?

I hope current racewalking clubs are flooded with new members and additional clubs spring up around the country. I want fitness racewalkers to become so common in our parks and on our sidewalks that no one pays them any more attention than they pay to the joggers the racewalkers speed past. I'd like demand for good racewalking shoes to be so high that the athletic shoe companies bring out new models specifically designed for racewalking. I want there to be more racewalking competitions so I'll have more races in which to participate, and I want more racewalking competitors so it will be more difficult for me to place in those races. Finally, I want you and me and many others to live longer, slimmer, healthier lives.

Throughout my career in and around state government, I've never been big on the "vision thing." I've been more of a nuts-and-bolts, get-things-done-correctly, kind of guy. But I do have a vision for baby boomers and racewalking. I see a time a few years into the future when the sport reaches the "tipping point" of popularity like jogging did in the 1960s. Hundreds or perhaps thousands of racewalkers will sign up for an event just as huge numbers of runners now sign up for road races and marathons. I envision fierce competition at the front of the races among a few elite competitors while the rest of us trail behind, enjoying the satisfaction of completing the race and reaping the health benefits of this fantastic sport.

You can enjoy racewalking the day you begin. But it will be a challenge for the rest of your life.

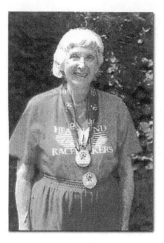

# Racewalker Profile

**Jean Brunnenkant**
Overland Park, KS
Year of Birth: 1916

During the first 75 years of her life, Jean Brunnenkant didn't know racewalking existed. This changed when she saw a contest at a local senior event. That was more than 15 years ago.

"With my background of teaching physical education and dance and with the fine help from the Heartland Racewalkers members, I learned the basic technique of racewalking," she said. "After about a year I was encouraged to enter the state senior Olympics in Topeka, Kansas, where one can qualify for the National Senior Games." Brunnenkant went to her first National Senior Games in 1993 and earned a gold medal in the 5K and a silver medal in the 1,500 meters in the 75-79 age group.

"I found it to be a challenge, along with some fun, to work on my technique and speed," she said. "Keeping a record of my walks helped me make racewalking a regular activity. I also used a stopwatch and a pacer watch to help improve my time."

Brunnenkant's training includes racewalking two or three miles five days a week, and she goes a longer distance of four or five miles once a week. Her consistent training paid off in competition. She went to three additional National Senior Games and won six more gold medals. Her most recent victories were in the 90-94 age group at the 2007 National Senior Games in Louisville, KY.

Brunnenkant suggested those contemplating racewalking consider the following benefits:

- You can do this sport any time of day or evening in any appropriate location.
- You need no equipment other than good shoes.
- You can do it alone or with companions.
- You can compete if you want.
- You take little risk of injury. (She's had only some foot/leg tendonitis.)
- Your heart and lungs will be grateful.

# Racewalker Profile

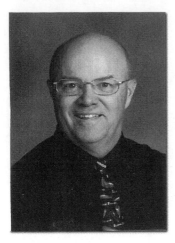

**William A. Riley, Jr.**
Belleville, IL
Year of Birth: 1953

Bill Riley began racewalking a few years ago when he could no longer run because of recurring knee problems. Now he trains five days a week at a local high school or park. He also works with a trainer once a month.

"I enjoy training in almost any weather," he said. "I draw the line at freezing rain and rain with lightning. Currently I alternate distance days of three to four miles where I stress stamina at speed with slower days of one to two miles where the emphasis is on technique. The technique days may also involve interval training with the major portion being 100 meter sprints," said Riley, who primarily competes in shorter events such as the 1500 meter racewalk.

Racewalking has given Riley more energy and his best fitness level ever. His resting pulse rate is 46 to 50 beats per minute, and he's trimmed up so much he's gotten a new wardrobe.

Riley earned several medals in area and state senior Olympics competitions and placed 7th in his age group in the 1,500 meter event at the 2007 National Senior Games in Louisville. He focuses on his time of completion in an event rather than where he places among the competitors. "My goal is to always finish under nine minutes," Riley said.

Riley has not had any injuries from racewalking – "just minor aches and pains associated with strenuous exercise – nothing that Biofreeze, ice or a massage won't fix," he said.

"Don't get discouraged when your shins complain loud and long when you start," Riley advised newcomers to racewalking. "You are just using muscles that you have never used before – it will pass."

# Chapter Two: What Is Racewalking?

USA Track & Field is the national governing body for track & field, long distance running and "race walking." Note that USATF refers to the sport with the two-word name "race walking," and I refer to the sport with the single word "racewalking." The world seems to be split on whether it's one word or two words. I prefer one word because I think when one sees the word "racewalking" it is clearly a reference to a specific sport while "race walking" could be interpreted as just walking fast. Regardless of the spelling of racewalking, the USATF defines what it is.

## The Two-Part Definition

The official definition, found in Rule 232 of the USATF Competition Rules, is:

> Race walking is a progression of steps so taken that the walker makes contact with the ground so that no visible (to the human eye) loss of contact occurs.
>
> The advancing leg must be straightened (i.e. not bent at the knee) from the moment of first contact with the ground until in the vertical upright position.

## The Contact-with-the-Ground Portion of the Definition

The first half of the definition would be self explanatory if it weren't for the words "visible (to the human eye)." This means that it must appear to a racewalking judge that at least one of a competitor's feet is always in contact with the ground. It must look like the front foot touches the ground before the back foot leaves the ground.

In practice, however, good racewalkers sometimes may have both feet off the ground for a fraction of a second each stride. If you slow or stop a video replay of a top walker, you may find a point where both feet are slightly airborne. But if you view the video in regular time, at least one foot appears to always be in contact with the ground.

I haven't had to worry about the first part of the definition yet. My feet spend too much time on the ground. Perhaps further training and improvement of my technique will increase my stride rate so that I will have to be concerned about being observably airborne.

Fast racewalkers do get called on this, though. When I finished the 2007 National Senior Games 1,500 meter racewalk I looked at my wife up in the stands and held up six fingers because I knew there were five contestants ahead of me. She shook her head and held up five fingers. I didn't realize that judges disqualified the competitor in second place coming down the home stretch on the final lap and pulled him off the track.

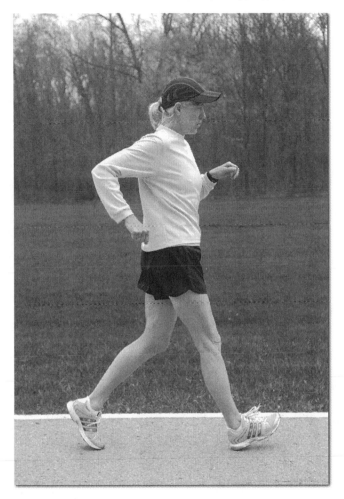

*Figure 2-1: Cathy Mayfield's lead foot clearly has made contact with the ground before her trailing foot has lost contact.*

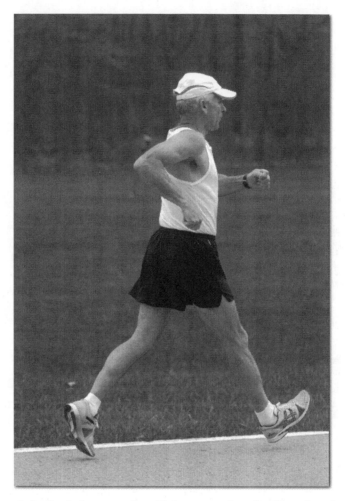

*Figure 2-2: Both feet may be off the ground and still within the legal definition if the loss of contact happens so quickly that the human eye cannot detect it in real time.*

## The Straightened-Leg Portion of the Definition

This rule, although it seems a bit odd to someone new to the sport, means exactly what it states. At the time the heel of your lead foot strikes the ground, you must have straightened your leg at the knee. You cannot bend your leg at the knee until your leg is vertical under your body. After your leg passes vertical, you may bend the knee.

The result is not the same as walking "stiff-legged" where you awkwardly swing the leg forward still straightened at the knee. In proper racewalking form, you bend your knee for your leg's forward movement and then straighten it again for the heel strike.

It is difficult to visualize the racewalking process from a mere explanation of the rules. The chapter on technique can assist the visualization, but watching someone racewalk is more helpful. Perhaps you could visit a local racewalking club, which you may locate through the Web sites in the Appendix.

You can watch video clips of Max Walker and Cathy Mayfield, who demonstrate racewalking techniques in the photos in this book, at http://www.boomerwalk.com. The North American Racewalking Foundation (NARF) Web site (http://www.philsport.com/narf/) has an excellent stick-figure animation of a racewalker and also has a video of a racewalker moving at an incredible pace. You may want to look at those now to give you a basic feel for the technique. You are referred to them again later in the book after a more complete discussion of technique enables you to better analyze what you are seeing.

Beginning racewalkers may find compliance with the USATF definition a bit awkward. I certainly did, and my form still suffers when I try to go at my fastest speed. When I walk at a moderate training pace, my gait feels natural and smooth. As I try to go faster, my form breaks down and my walking begins to feels rough. So my advice – and the advice seems to be the same from every experienced racewalker I encounter – is to start walking at a slow or moderate speed, concentrating on your form. As your technique improves and you feel more comfortable, add to your speed.

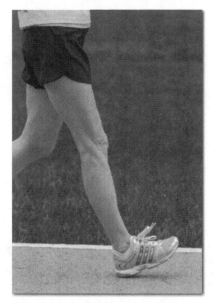 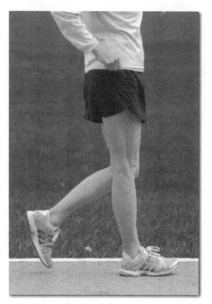

*Figure 2-3: The lead leg must be straightened at the knee by the time the heel contacts the ground.*

*Figure 2-4: The leg must remain straightened at the knee from the moment of contact until the leg is vertical under the body.*

# A Short History of Racewalking[8]

In the late 16th and early 17th century English aristocrats used "footmen" to accompany their coaches as the gentry traveled about the countryside. A footman's duties included hurrying ahead of the coach as it approached an inn or country estate so the staff would be prepared for the aristocrats' arrival. Gambling was popular among the wealthy during that period, and the aristocrats began to wager large amounts on races among their footmen.

Footmen were expected to keep up with a coach without running using a process described as "fair heel and toe." However, the footmen were "allowed to trot, as necessary, to ward off cramp."

In the second half of the 18th century races against time grew more popular. The participants, called "pedestrians," earned significant prize money for reaching a goal such as walking 100 miles in less than 24 hours (and

---

[8] *Information for this history of racewalking is from "A Brief History of Racewalking in the United States," an article by Phil Howell on the Web site of the North American Racewalking Foundation (http://www.philsport.com/narf/). Howell's article was first published in Walk Talk, the newsletter of the Walking Club of Georgia, and was based upon a dissertation by the late William Gordon Wallace titled "Racewalking in America: Past and Present." Permission for the use of this material granted by Phil Howell.*

earning the title "Centurion") or walking one mile each hour for 1,000 consecutive hours. The latter event lasted 41 days and 16 hours.

In the early 19$^{th}$ century racing between men reemerged, and, bolstered by gambling, became the most popular sport in England. America also embraced walking races, and up to 25,000 onlookers came to witness competitions. Pedestrianism grew in popularity until shortly before the Civil War and then took off again after the war. A 1,136 mile race from Portland, Maine, to Chicago in 1867 paid the winner $10,000.

Towns around the country built walking stadiums and indoor tracks. Champions from England and America competed on each other's soil. Races among women became popular as well. The "Long Distance Championship of the World" race in 1888, a highly successful, six-day event, actually helped bring about the decline of pedestrianism. The rules allowed the athletes to "go-as-you-please," and running took over.

Amateur competitions, which frequently included walking events, developed contemporaneously in private athletic clubs and colleges. The Amateur Athletic Union (AAU) formed in the late 1880s, and the International Olympic Committee (IOC) followed in 1893. The first modern Olympic Games in 1896 did not include a walking race. The 1904 Olympic games included an 800-yard walk as a component of the "all-rounder" event, the predecessor of the decathlon. The racewalk was an independent event at the non-recognized 1906 Intercalated Olympic Games and has been a separate event at every official Olympic Games since 1908.

U.S. racewalkers were somewhat successful in the 1920 Olympics, but interest in the sport soon dwindled here and abroad. Henry Laskau rekindled some interest in the United States at mid-century, and other American racewalkers gained attention in the 1960s. The advent of masters track and field competition in the late 1960s brought out older racewalkers.

In 1977 American Todd Scully became the first racewalker to accomplish the long-sought goal of a six-minute mile. Interest and accomplishments grew worldwide during the 1980s, highlighted at the Seoul Olympics in 1988, where 28 racewalkers surpassed the 1984 records. In 1992 the Olympics added a racewalking event for women. Improved facilities, training and coaching enhanced the performance of U.S. athletes in recent years.

Both the rules for racewalking and the rulemaking body for amateur sport changed a few times during the 1900s. Early in the century authorities added a requirement that the knee be straightened at some point during a stride. In the 1970s a rule modification provided the knee must not be bent when directly under the body. The Athletics Congress (TAC/USA) superceded the AAU in 1979, and TAC/USA was renamed USA Track & Field (USATF) in 1992. In 1996 rule makers adopted the current requirements that the leg must not be bent at the knee from the moment of first contact with the ground until in the vertical upright position and that there be no loss of contact visible "to the human eye."

# Racewalker Profile

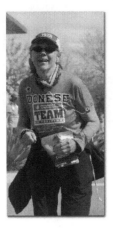

**Donese Mayfield**
Albuquerque, NM
Year of Birth: 1946

Donese Mayfield recently joined the New Mexico Racewalkers Club to work on her speed and racewalking technique. Before that she power walked, and she only began that a little more than a year ago.

"I am not an athlete," Mayfield said. "I'm a therapeutic musician. I play music for hospice patients. A doctor asked me to go see a 34-year-old, single mom who was dying of leukemia. That experience led me to sign up to walk a marathon with Team in Training, a part of the Leukemia and Lymphoma Society. They teach people how to do events such as marathons, half marathons, triathalons, et cetera. In return you raise money for blood cancer research. Training for the marathon and completing it was such a terrific experience that I wanted to continue in the sport."

In an 11-month period this "nonathlete" completed a marathon, two half marathons and a 5K race. "The experience has been an absolute win-win for me," she said. "I enjoy the experience. I am healthier, have lower blood pressure, sleep better and have gotten other family members involved. I tell them that if their mom can complete a marathon when she is 60, they can get their anatomy moving, too."

Mayfield is realistic about exercise. "I am 61 years old. There are going to be body parts that hurt and don't work like they did 10, 20 or 30 years ago. That's just the way it is. So I have started religiously stretching after I walk and doing yoga every week to stay flexible. These aches and pains are not going to prevent me from walking and enjoying this sport. I just work around them."

Mayfield's tips for beginners include:

- The hardest part of training is putting on your shoes and walking out the door.
- There's no need for speed. Just get out the door and do it.
- Find a walking buddy.

# Racewalker Profile

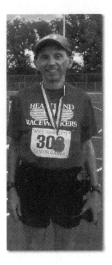

**Alan Poisner, M.D.**
Overland Park, KS
Year of Birth: 1934

Dr. Alan Poisner developed sciatic pain after three years of running. He visited a local racewalking group and was attracted to the sport because it offered the same fitness, competition and social opportunities he enjoyed in local road races without the injuries he sustained running. That was more than 20 years ago.

Poisner was a founding member of the Heartland Racewalkers, a club that meets weekly, sponsors clinics and promotes racewalking in the media. "Our club provides an educational experience for our members beyond racewalking since we have talks on other health-related issues," he said. "We also stress flexibility with stretching at our clinics, something that many would have difficulty doing on their own."

Poisner trains about five days a week. When he is training for one of the two half-marathons he racewalks each year, he averages about 30 miles a week with a long walk of 10-12 miles. Otherwise he walks about 22 miles a week with a long walk of 5-6 miles. Poisner won gold medals in state, national and international competitions.

"I cannot claim any weight loss because I was slim when I began racewalking," he said. "But my cardiovascular system has improved as attested to by the decrease in my resting heart rate and an increase in stamina that permitted me to walk two marathons.

"The only injury that I have had (from racewalking) that necessitated seeing a professional was in the early years when I injured my shoulder and developed bursitis because I was keeping my shoulders raised instead of down and relaxed," he said.

"I tell my new members there are two rules," he said. "One, don't hurt yourself – injury prevention – and, two, have fun – the basis for life-long activity. Also, for those who may want to enter competitive events, I suggest patience in developing speed with emphasis on technique. I kept getting faster for eight years after I began racewalking."

# Chapter Three: What Equipment Do You Need?

One of the great features of racewalking is that it doesn't take a lot of ancillary paraphernalia. Whether you are just in it for the exercise or you are competing on the national level, you don't need to go out and spend a lot on the latest high tech gear. A pair of proper shoes gets you started. This may be a disappointment for those boomer consumers among us who find gratification in buying the largest titanium drivers for our golf bags or the lightest carbon framesets for our bicycles.

I was surprised to discover that the shoes most of us have for running, jogging or knocking around are not the best shoes for racewalking. Most running shoes have thick, cushioned heels to absorb the shock of pounding on the pavement. But racewalking is a smooth, low-impact activity. You don't need the cushion to protect your joints. In fact, the thick heel makes it more difficult to execute proper racewalking form.

You may find a few shoes designed specifically for racewalking, but not many. Some racewalkers use running shoes with little cushioning, known as racing flats. I wear size 15 shoes, so that limits my choice. I went to the local running store, looked at the various styles and found the one with the lowest heel the store could order in my size.

The front half of the soles of racewalking shoes should be flexible. When you push off to propel yourself forward, this added flexibility promotes efficiency.

As with all athletic shoes, racewalking shoes should have sufficient arch support. I wear custom orthotic inserts in my everyday shoes and also in my racewalking shoes.

Other important features of a good racewalking shoe are that they have a roomy toe box as well as a sturdy heel cup. A final thought: it is best to shop for shoes at the end of the day because your feet may swell a bit.

The racewalking Web sites generally have sections about racewalking shoes. It's a major topic among racewalkers – partly because there isn't any other equipment to talk about and partly because the shoe companies frequently drop or modify their models. If boomers take up the sport in numbers, shoe companies will rush to make us the shoes we need.

In the meantime if you can't find anything satisfactory and have some extra money, Hersey Custom Shoe Company (www.herseycustomshoe.com) of Fitchburg, MA, makes two models of custom-fit racewalking shoes. Hersey's competition model has been used by some U.S. Olympians. The shoes are expensive, and the company has a backlog of several months.

If you racewalk in competition, you will need shorts that give the judges a sufficient view of the knee to ascertain whether it is straightened properly. Most of my exercise shorts are the newer style that graze the top of my knees. They are not appropriate for racewalk competition. I had to dig through several layers in my chest of drawers to find some old shorts that stopped several inches above my knee.

In cold weather judges may allow you to wear tights that cover your legs, but the tights must be form fitting so that judges have a good view of whether your knee is straightened. You can't wear sweat pants or jogging suit pants in competition because they do not provide an adequate view of the leg. Of course, when you are training you can wear as many layers as you need for comfort.

On cool days I wear a hat and cloth gloves, and on cold days I add something to cover my ears. Modern moisture-wicking materials help move perspiration away from your body to keep you warmer on cold days and cooler on hot days.

The other piece of equipment I use is a heart rate monitor. It consists of a sensor on an elastic band I wear around my chest and a watch-like receiver for my wrist. I purchased a no-frills model for about $50. It gives me a good sense of how much I am working my body at any time. You can certainly racewalk without a heart rate monitor, but I find it useful to me as I train. It also helps me evaluate my effort in relation to the level suggested in *Younger Next Year*.

That's about it for equipment. You probably can get started without buying a thing.

# Racewalker Profile

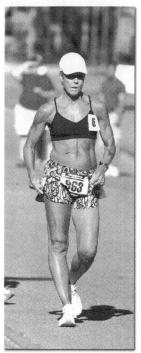

**Lynn Tracy**
Racine, WI
Year of Birth: 1952

After 20 years as a competitive softball and volleyball player, Lynn Tracy suffered injuries and arthritis that prevented her from keeping up with younger players. But her maladies didn't prevent her from walking fast. She began timing herself walking routes in her neighborhood and read some books about racewalking. In the winter she walked in a mall until one night a security guard warned her to slow down or she would be evicted or arrested. Tracy needed a new place to walk and after a search discovered coach Mike DeWitt of the University of Wisconsin-Parkside and the Parkside Athletic Club. The racewalking club has grown from 6 members to more than 30 since she joined in 1990.

"Everybody is incredibly supportive of one another – whether we're walking a 14-minute or 8-minute mile," she said. "The camaraderie is what keeps people coming back week after week. Even during our darkest times, club mates are always there for us. They provide shoulders to cry on, cheerleaders for our best efforts and competition during our weekly workouts and local trial walks."

Tracy has experienced some dark times. She's had several major non-racewalking-related surgeries, the most recent a mastectomy for breast cancer. But she's also had many shining times. She's an eight-time national champion and in October 2007, less than a year after her cancer surgery, set an American record for the 55-59 age group at the USA Track and Field 5K nationals.

"The health benefits of racewalking are incredible." Tracy said. "At 55 people are constantly amazed by my enthusiastic energy with everything I do. I have lost about 12 pounds, toned my entire body (Tracy also started lifting weights.), and am leaner and in better shape and condition than I have ever been. I feel more confident and empowered since I started racewalking and winning competitions."

In her first year of racewalking Tracy injured a hamstring. She attributes the injury to going too fast too soon. She continued racing, and the injury bothered her for a long time.

"Nowadays, I listen to my body," she said, "and if something hurts I actually take it easy for a few days. I get a complete body/sports massage regularly. In other words, I treat myself better rather than beating myself up."

Tracy suggested that as a new racewalker you should:

- Concentrate on technique rather than speed to become more efficient and faster.
- Find a good coach and watch videotapes of yourself.
- Judge yourself on your own merits, not according to how fast others walk.
- Keep a workout log so you can see how far you have progressed.
- Remember to have fun!

# Racewalker Profile

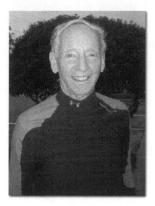

**Charles M. Williams**
Atlanta, GA
Year of Birth: 1931

Charles M. Williams took up racewalking in 2005 after he injured his knee running. He learned the form and skills from the Walking Club of Georgia and became an avid proponent of the sport.

"I'm trying to get older runners to switch over to racewalking before they disintegrate from injuries. I tend to pass too many of my old teammates on half marathons these days. They are suffering from a variety of ailments and seem to be feverishly trying to finish one more race before things come to an abrupt halt. I'm not opposed to running, but getting personal records at something new in my advancing years has done wonders for my outlook on life."

Williams encourages racewalking in area high schools and works with adults, too. "I've been a volunteer racewalk coach for Team in Training marathon and half marathon participants – mostly overweight, age-40-plus women, who are trying to lose a few pounds," he said. "An appreciable number succeed."

He has not experienced any injuries from racewalking, but he has noticed the benefits. "My posture has remarkably improved," he said. "Aches and pains have melted away."

Williams trains four days a week, and his sessions range from speed work of two or three miles to distance work of more than nine miles. His efforts have paid off with places at USATF National Masters and National Senior Games.

"Pay attention to form before trying for speed," Williams suggested. "Get a good coach – minor changes in form can yield major improvements in performance."

36

# Chapter Four: What Do You Need to Know about Technique?

In the spring of 2007 my son and I met in Florida to see a few spring training baseball games. I knew that Florida was an active area for racewalking so I checked the racewalking Web sites before I left for the trip to see if any races were scheduled while I would be there. It turned out the Henry Laskau Memorial Florida State 5K Racewalk Championship was scheduled within a half hour's drive of where we would be staying. I emailed the race director for details so I could observe the race and was surprised when he said I was welcome to participate.

I went to the race intending to watch, but I wore walking clothes in case I decided to take part. When I got there the race director again asked if I wanted to participate. At that time I wasn't a member of USA Track and Field so I wouldn't be eligible for an award. However, I could still walk, get a T-shirt and be in a judged race where my form would be monitored. What other sport would allow a last minute walk-on to participate in a state championship?

Henry Laskau's son was the official starter for the race. At the time the name Henry Laskau didn't mean anything to me. But in his book, *Racewalk Like a Champion*, Jeff Salvage provides an extensive biography on Laskau and other notable racewalkers. Laskau was a top middle distance runner in Germany who escaped from a Nazi labor camp, came to the United States and took up racewalking. In the 1940s and 1950s Laskau represented the United States in the Olympics three times, won 43 national titles and held many American records. In 1951 he set a then world record of 6 minutes and 12.2 seconds for one mile at Madison Square Garden. Salvage refers to Laskau as "the Dean of American racewalkers." He died in 2000 at age 83.

The race was the longest I had attempted at the time, and I was happy to finish with no red cards for form violations. I finished ahead of a few walkers but behind several men considerably older than I.

After the race Frank Alongi offered an informal clinic. Alongi was a distance runner on the Italian Olympic team in 1948 and 1952. His brother was a racewalker, and Alongi, an engineer, did his doctoral dissertation on the biomechanics of racewalking. He came to the United States in the mid-1950s and has spent much of his free time here coaching racewalkers and encouraging the sport.

Alongi demonstrated the technique for us in slow motion. The heel of his front foot made contact with the ground not too far in front of his body. He had straightened his leg at the knee and flexed his ankle so that the toe of his shoe pointed upward. As his body moved forward and his leg became vertical under his body, he rocked forward from his heel to the sole of his foot. The toe of his shoe still pointed upward. The bottom of his foot was like the curved runner on the bottom of a rocking chair. As his body continued to move forward and his leg trailed behind, his foot rocked forward onto his toes and his heel began to rise off the ground. At this point he extended his ankle and pushed off with his toes to give his body a forward thrust.

The following four figures show the motion of the foot throughout the stride in racewalking as demonstrated to me by Frank Alongi.

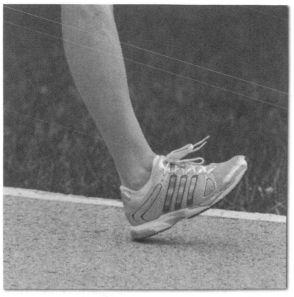

*Figure 4-1: The ankle and the toe of the shoe are flexed upward at the heel strike.*

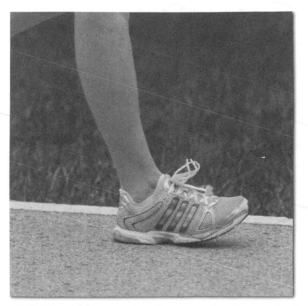

*Figure 4-2: The ankle remains flexed as the foot rocks forward and the sole makes contact with the ground.*

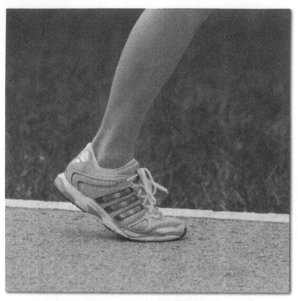

*Figure 4-3: The heel begins to lift off the ground as the leg trails behind.*

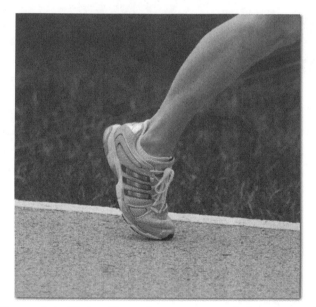

*Figure 4-4: The ankle and toe are extended to thrust the body forward as the foot loses contact with the ground.*

This is much different than running or jogging. When you run or jog, your body endures a jolt at the time of the heel strike. The force of the heel strike tends to cause your ankle to extend downward, and the sole of your foot may slap against the pavement. Because there is much less force on your heel strike in racewalking, you can keep your ankle flexed with the toe pointing up as you rock forward onto the sole of your foot. The lower heel of a good shoe for racewalking helps you execute this form. The thicker heel of a typical running shoe increases the height of the rest of the foot off the ground at the time of the heel strike and makes it more difficult to hold the ankle in the flexed upward position through the rocking process.

## Short Stride in Front, Long Stride in Back

Before I began racewalking I walked a lot on a treadmill at the local fitness club. When I wanted to increase my speed, I would just turn up the speed on the treadmill and take longer and longer steps, reaching my front leg farther and farther forward. I'm 6'5" tall so I can cover quite a bit of ground with a stretched-out stride.

But that's not the way it works with racewalking. The second part of the definition of racewalking requires you to straighten your leg at the knee when your heel strikes the ground in front of you. It's easy to visualize what happens when you stretch a straightened leg way out in front of you as your body is moving forward. The leg acts as a brake that tries to stop your forward motion. In order to go forward your body has to vault up and over the stiff leg.

However, if the heel of your lead leg strikes the ground only slightly in front of your body, the braking effort is minimized and your body glides forward over the top of the straightened leg with little resistance. Some suggest the proper stride is approximately 30 percent in front of the body and 70 percent behind the body. That is a goal I'd like to work toward, but I'm not very flexible, and it will be a while before I get there.

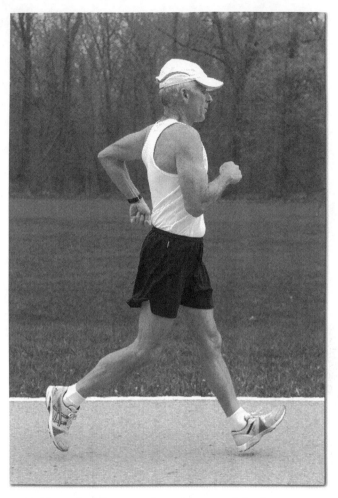

*Figure 4-5: Note the short stride in front and the long stride in back.*

## Toe of Shoe Up

In my description of Frank Alongi's demonstration, I talked about the toe of his shoe pointing upward. Flexing your foot at the ankle and pointing the toe of your shoe upward helps ensure that you have your leg straightened at the knee. Keep the toe of your shoe pointed up as you rock forward on your foot and you will be less likely to get a red card for a bent knee. **Note:** Do not try to raise your toes through the top of your shoes. The toe of your shoe is pointed up primarily because you are flexing your ankle and not because you are raising your toes inside your shoes.

For many people new to racewalking, a most difficult aspect is to keep their ankles flexed and toes of their shoes pointing upward. The muscles that enable you to flex your ankle upward are located on the front of your legs just outside your shin bones. Racewalking newcomers will find these muscles tire quickly and will start to burn after walking a short distance. When my daughter was in college and regularly was running three miles on a treadmill, she tried racewalking with me for the first time. She could racewalk only about 50 yards before the muscles on the fronts of her shins gave out.

Fortunately, the muscles on the front of the legs that flex the ankles upward strengthen quickly. They will get stronger as you practice more. You can add some exercises to bring them along more quickly. (See Chapter Six.) As with all new physical activities, you should ease into it. Don't push yourself too much at first so that the soreness remains even after the workout. You don't want to get so sore that you have to stop for a few days. Remember, you have the rest of your life to work on this skill.

As I described earlier, a good racewalking shoe has a lower heel than the thick cushioning found on most running and cross-training shoes. You will find it easier to keep your ankle flexed and toe up if you have a shoe with a lower heel. I started with some old running shoes with very thick heels, and it made a significant difference when I switched to lower-heeled shoes.

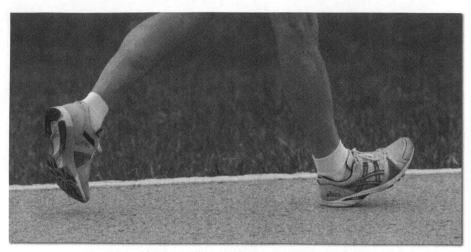

*Figure 4-6: At heel contact the ankle should be flexed*
*causing the toe of the shoe to point up.*

## Hip Motion

In past decades racewalking technique emphasized the push off with the toe as the major thrust that propels the body forward. According to Jeff Salvage, current thought is that the hips are the driving force forward.

Your hip pivots or rotates forward in conjunction with the forward movement of your leg. For example, your right hip thrusts forward as your right leg comes forward. Your right foot plants on the ground, and then your body moves forward over and past your right leg as your left hip thrusts forward with your left leg.

The benefit of this motion, often referred to as "hip rotation," is easy to understand. Assume your hips didn't pivot and your stride was 30 inches long. Now assume you can move the right side of your hips two inches in front of your body with the right leg for the heel strike and the right side of your hips trails two inches behind your body by the time your toes are pushing off the ground behind you. You have just added four inches to your stride. Four inches may not seem like much, but if you multiply that by thousands of steps, you are significantly increasing your distance traveled with the same number of steps.

The pelvis isn't very flexible so when you thrust your right hip forward from behind your body to in front of your body, the outside of your hip actually traces a slight arc out and then back in. Assume a racewalker is walking on a straight line painted on the pavement. If you look down from above, as the right hip is thrust from behind the body to in front of the body, you will see the outside of the hip move in an arc slightly further from the painted line as the hip catches up with the body and then move closer to the painted line as the hip continues in front of the body. This is not a swiveling of the hips from side to side; it is just a slight arc that is a function of the pelvis pivoting on a center point.

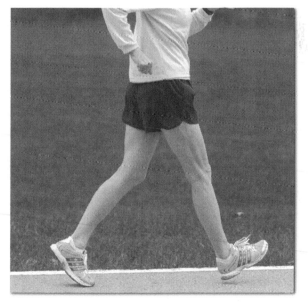

*Figure 4-7: The hip should pivot forward with the lead leg.*
*This hip rotation increases the length of the stride.*

In addition to the hip rotation, the hip also tilts slightly up and down through the course of a complete stride. The following two diagrams illustrate the proper hip motion. If you view a racewalker from the right side and you focus on a point on the outside of the right hip as the racewalker walks from left to right, the path taken by the point on the side of the hip is shown in Figure 4-8 and Figure 4-9. Both figures show key phases of the racewalking stride.

Figure 4-8 illustrates the path the point on the hip travels when a racewalker walks on a road or track. From the time of heel strike (1 on the left of Figure 4-8) until the leg is vertical under the body (2), the point moves up. As the body moves forward and the leg trails behind, the point on the side of the hip moves down through the toe off behind the body (3) and continues to move down as the bent leg begins to swing forward. This is referred to as "hip drop." When the bent leg swings past vertical beneath the body (4), the point begins to move up again and returns to the same level as the starting point at heel strike (1 on the right of Figure 4-8).

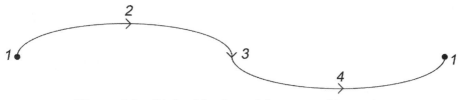

*Figure 4-8 – Right side view of the proper hip motion when racewalking on a road*

Figure 4-9 illustrates the path the point on the hip travels when a racewalker walks on a treadmill. In fact you can see a video of this process on Salvage's *Race Walk Like a Champion* DVD. Keep in mind that when walking on a treadmill the trunk of the body doesn't move. Instead, the belt on the treadmill moves beneath the body. At the time of heel strike (1) the hip is pivoted forward so the point on the side of the hip is in front of the body. As the moving belt brings the leg to vertical under the body (2), the point on the hip moves back toward the center of the body and also moves upward. As the belt moves the leg further behind the body, the point on the hip moves behind the body and moves downward. After toe off (3), the racewalker begins to swing the bent leg forward, bringing the point on the hip forward at the same time. The point on the hip moves down until the bent leg passes under the body (4). Then, as the leg and hip continue to move forward, the point on the side of the hip moves up until it returns to the original position at heel strike.

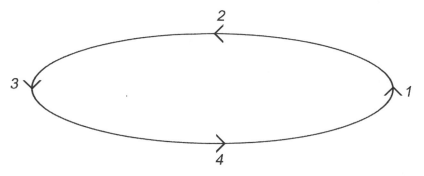

*Figure 4-9 – Right side view of the proper hip motion*
*when racewalking on a treadmill*

Dave McGovern points out that the amount of hip movement in racewalkers varies depending upon the flexibility of the individuals. Some people are hyperflexible and exhibit lots of hip movement. Others have much less. Over time you will discover what amount of hip movement works for you.

I expect a continuing discussion among racewalkers about how much of the forward motion is driven by the hip flexors thrusting the leg forward and how much comes from the push off by the trailing foot. My conversations with racewalkers indicate that the relative amount from each source varies from racewalker to racewalker. As a new racewalker you should be aware that both can contribute to your forward motion, and you should pay attention to both as you learn the technique. Each of us has our own physical characteristics. With experience and, I hope, with the help of others, you will find the balance that works best for you.

## Foot Placement

Visualize yourself walking down the middle of a sidewalk with your normal gait. Assume a painted line the width of a striping line on a highway runs down the middle of that sidewalk. As you imagine yourself walking down the sidewalk normally, you probably will see your right foot fall off to the right of the line and your left foot fall off to the left of the line. Your weight shifts to your right foot on one side of the line with one step and then to your left foot on the other side of the line with the next step.

In contrast, a racewalker's feet land on the line down the middle of the sidewalk. This is a function of the arc of the racewalker's hip motion. Assume again that you are looking down on the racewalker from above. As the trailing foot is about to leave the ground, that side of the hip is pivoted behind the body, the outside of the hip is close to the centerline and the foot is on the centerline. As the hip is thrust forward, the outside of the hip moves away from the centerline and carries the leg out with it until the hip and leg are even with the body. As the hip and leg move in front of the body, the outside of the hip arcs in toward the centerline and carries the leg with it until the foot falls on the centerline in front of the racewalker. The body moves efficiently forward without the lost energy of the side to side movement of a regular walking gait.

For some racewalkers the footfall will land on the center of the three- or four-inch wide line. For others the hip action may not bring the foot all the way to the middle of the line, but the foot will touch the outside of the line. The racewalker's center of gravity moves directly forward rather than moving from side to side as is does in a normal walking gait.

This is easy to practice. When you are walking pick out a straight line in the walking surface such as a painted stripe in an empty parking lot. Pivot your hips so that every footstep touches that line.

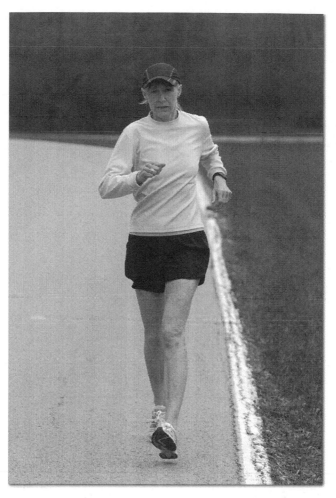

*Figure 4-10: The foot should land near the centerline in front of the body so the walker moves straight forward and does not bob side to side.*

## Arm Motion

The arms play an important part in proper racewalking technique. First, you need to know how to carry your arms and shoulders. Then it's important to understand their proper motion. I'm still learning and working on this.

Several observers have cautioned me about carrying my shoulders too high. I tend to tighten them and pull them up around my neck, especially when I am trying to increase my speed. That's not the way to do it. Relax your shoulders. Let them hang down or you'll waste a lot of needless energy trying to keep them raised. I sometimes still catch my shoulders tight and up around my neck when I'm in a race pushing for more speed.

If you walk with your relaxed, normal stride, you will notice that your arms naturally swing in counterbalance with the position of your legs. As your right leg comes forward, your right arm swings backward. Your right foot plants on the ground and then, as your body moves forward over your right leg, your right arm swings forward to counterbalance the position of the leg.

The motion is the same in racewalking, although the movement is exaggerated. Your hands go forward to approximately mid-chest height and should be comfortably in front of the centerline of your body. On the backswing your hands go a couple of inches further back than your hips and should pass close to your hip rather than flailing out to your side. Don't overdo the distance your arms move. You've undoubtedly seen some "power walkers" striding along, pumping their fists forward and up as high as their heads and backward a foot behind their bodies. That is inefficient and not good racewalking form.

During a senior Olympics race Patricia Beam, a racewalker and fabulous multi-sport senior athlete who is profiled later in this book, yelled at me from the track sidelines. "Bend your elbows. Short levers!" she coached.

I knew my arms should be bent at about a right angle at the elbow. I didn't realize that over time I had begun to carry them much straighter than that. The next day I concentrated on keeping my elbows bent more, and I could immediately tell the difference in the cadence of my footsteps.

Beam's comment about "short levers" made sense. If a grandfather clock is running too slowly, you adjust the speed by shortening the pendulum a bit. By bending my elbows more, I was

50

shortening the pendulum of my swinging arms and enabling them to move through a complete to-and-fro cycle faster. Since legs move in concert with arm swing, my stride was quicker, too.

The 90-degree angle bend at the elbows is an approximation and varies from individual to individual. The angle is correct when your shoulders are relaxed and your arms move through their full cycle of motion with the least effort. The angle of the bend at your elbow does not change during the cycle.

Don't waste energy clenching your fists. Just hold your hands in a relaxed curl. On a recent trip to the Boston area I went to a Tuesday evening session of the racewalking group from the Cambridge Sports Union at Harvard's track. Ken Mattsson, a 20-year racewalker and 10-year coach, suggested that one imagine holding a potato chip within one's closed hand without crushing it. This seems to work for me. If I concentrate on relaxed hands, my shoulders seem to relax, too.

Somewhere I got the incorrect idea that the shoulders were supposed to have a significant back and forth motion to accentuate the arm movement. I recently spent a couple of hours in a private lesson with coach Bonnie Stein. She quickly identified several problems with my upper body movement, including my exaggerated shoulder action. I later checked my Salvage and McGovern books and found Stein was exactly right – the arms swing in the shoulder sockets like a hinge. The experts also emphasize that the force of the back swing of the arm helps propel you forward – Newton's third law of motion (For every action there is an equal and opposite reaction.) at work.

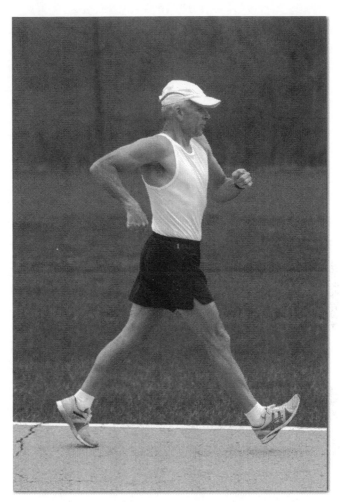

*Figure 4-11: As the leg and hip go forward, the arm swings backward. Note the elbow bent about 90 degrees and the hand not going much past the body.*

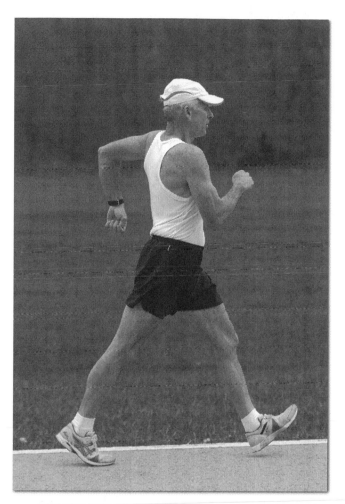

*Figure 4-12: As the leg trails behind the body, the arm swings forward with the hand only going to mid-chest height a comfortable distance in front of the body.*

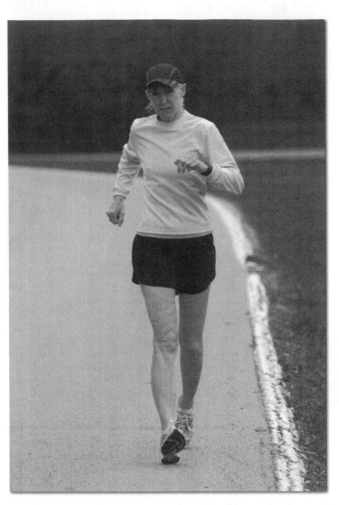

*Figure 4-13: The hand should travel to near the centerline of the chest. Note the relaxed shoulders and hands.*

## Posture

As a racewalker you should maintain an upright posture with head up and eyes looking forward. Don't slouch, lean forward or bend at the waist. If you remember 1996 Olympic 200-meter champion Michael Johnson's upright stature as he blazed down the track, you have the picture. At the Cambridge Sports Union session Mattsson demonstrated how standing upright with a high center of gravity makes one less stable and thus enables one to move forward with less effort.

## Putting It All Together

You need to keep several different aspects of technique in mind when beginning: knee straight, toe up, push off, hip pivoting, upright posture, eyes looking ahead, arm bent at the appropriate angle, and arm moving back as the hip is thrust forward. It will help if you actually watch someone do this. Unfortunately, racewalking doesn't (yet) get much coverage on television. You might see some video very late at night during the Olympics every four years.

If you have a club nearby, contact the club and arrange a visit where the members likely will be pleased to demonstrate the technique and help you learn it. The technique section of Jeff Salvage's Web site http://www.racewalk.com) includes a series of still photos of Jefferson Perez, an Olympic gold medalist and three-time world champion, that capture the details of the proper form. This would be a good time to revisit the video at http://www.boomerwalk.com and the stick figure animation and video at http://www.philsport.com/narf/ recommended in Chapter Two. By this point you have a better appreciation of the technique, and you can see how the elements fit together fluidly. The video of the racewalker on the NARF Web site actually was constructed using the series of still photos of Jefferson Perez that appear on Salvage's Web site. Finally, the Web sites in this book's Appendix identify racewalking videos and DVDs that are available to help you move up the learning curve.

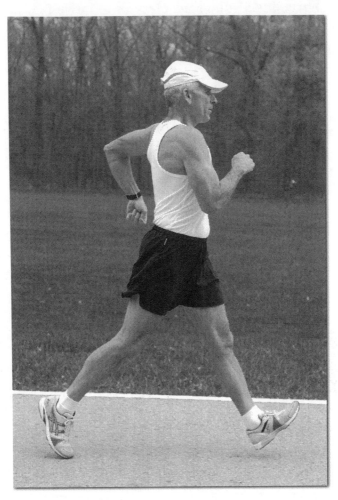

*Figure 4-14: This is the same photo as in the Introduction showing Max Walker in full stride exhibiting proper form. Note the following aspects of racewalking technique: The body is erect with the head up and looking forward. The ankle of the lead foot is flexed with the toe pointing upward and the knee is straightened. The ankle and toe of the trailing foot are extended to thrust the body forward. The stride is shorter in front and longer in back. The hip is pivoted forward with the lead leg, and the arm on that side of the body is back. The arms are bent about 90 degrees with the hand on the lead-leg side of the body going back just behind the body and the hand on the trailing-leg side of the body going to mid-chest height.*

## Practice, Practice, Practice

The form seems awkward and the gait a bit rough at first, but practice makes it smoother. At the Dave McGovern clinic I attended one of the young women attendees is a potential future Olympian. Her form is a beautiful thing to watch. The movement of her legs and feet is as fluid as one pedaling a bicycle. When you have the opportunity to observe really good racewalkers, take special note of their heads. The racewalkers are flying along, but their heads are not bobbing up and down a bit.

The technique comes more easily to some than to others. A couple of middle-aged women at the McGovern clinic had good form, and I think they had started racewalking only a few months before. It didn't come that easy for me. After three years, my racewalking form feels more natural, but when I try to speed up my leg turnover in a short race such as the 1,500 meters, I again feel the roughness in my gait.

It helps to have someone observe you walking. After watching me in a competition, my wife said, "Everyone else walks upright, but you walk bent over." She didn't even know what to look for, and still she gave me some help in correcting my form.

It's best to get help from other racewalkers early on before bad habits are ingrained in your muscle memory. If you can join a club or get some other walkers to train with you, you can help each other with your form.

If you have access to a video camera, have someone take a video of you racewalking. You may also do it yourself with a video camera and tripod. Position the camera so you get a side view as you walk by. Also shoot some video walking on a straight line toward the camera. Review the video at regular speed and at a slow speed or frame by frame. Check your posture to make certain you are upright and looking forward, not at your feet. Make sure the toe on your lead foot is up and your leg is not bent at the knee. Look to see if you are pushing off with your back foot. Examine the movement of your shoulders, arms and hips. Finally, see if there is ever a time when both feet are off the ground. In the video taken while walking toward the camera, make sure your feet are landing on the line and not shifting from one side of the line to the other.

Once you get some feedback, put the information to work improving your technique. It takes repetition to train your body and make the technique a fluid, natural movement so practice, practice, practice.

# Racewalker Profile

**Sandy Lawson**
Carmel, IN
Year of Birth: 1955

In 2005 Sandy Lawson entered a racewalk event and finished with a good time. Unfortunately, she was disqualified because she didn't use the proper technique. She wanted to learn the requirements and how she could go even faster so she joined the Indiana Racewalkers' Club.

"At the time I joined the club had trainers at every meeting who helped with form and speed work and answered any questions I had," she said. "Also, they were very encouraging, helpful and warm."

Lawson trains once a week at a university facility with the club and four days on her own at home. She varies her distances according to a training schedule geared to upcoming races.

She has racewalked in club races, local running/walking races and half marathons. "I have achieved my goal for this year of breaking a 10-minute mile in a 5K," she added.

Lawson's had some knee, hip flexor and hamstring problems, but she termed them "minor ailments" that responded to simple treatments.

Her advice to newcomers to the sport is "Stick with it; it will pay off."

# Racewalker Profile

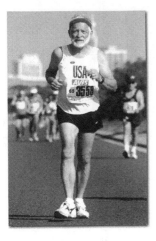

**Ryszard Nawrocki**
Rio Rancho, NM
Year of Birth: 1928

Ryszard Nawrocki began running in 1978 and completed 20 marathons. While living in Michigan in the mid-1980s he encountered a group of racewalkers led by Frank Alongi, the well-known racewalking coach. Nawrocki took up racewalking and for several years continued both running and racewalking. "In the early 1990s I switched to racewalking only," he said. "(It was) easier on my joints, and I was getting better results."

Nawrocki moved to New Mexico in 1994 after retirement and joined the New Mexico Racewalkers, Inc. He trains five or six times per week in season and less during the winter. His training racewalks vary from two to eight miles, and he does interval training on a track.

Nawrocki competes locally, nationally and internationally. He participated in nine biennial World Association of Veteran Athletes (now World Masters Athletics) Championships including events held in Finland, South Africa, England, Australia, Puerto Rico and Spain. Three times he was the second American finisher on the team that won the gold medal in the 20K team competition. He also is a certified USATF official and racewalking judge.

"Racewalking and training for it contributes greatly to my good health, well being and satisfaction in life," Nawrocki said. "It helps control my weight," he added. He suffered injuries in his running years, but now "only has occasional aches and pains after hard training or races." He advised those new to the sport to "get good instruction as to technique and training regimen," and to "train regularly but first in moderation until well conditioned."

# Chapter Five: Where Can You Walk?

When I started racewalking I did most of my training on a treadmill at home or at a fitness club. Winter in central Illinois often dictates a treadmill as my only alternative. Unfortunately, I picked up three bad habits by beginning on a treadmill without proper understanding of racewalking form.

The first habit, and one that continues to be the most difficult for me to break, is looking down toward my feet as I walk. I think it came from looking at the readout of speed, distance and heart rate on the treadmill's instrument panel. Part of it, I'm sure, came from looking to see if my knee was straight and my toes were up once I knew that was part of racewalking form.

"Keep your head up," Patricia Beam called from the side of the track when she saw me in my first racewalk competition. (I'd be a lot better racewalker if I lived closer to Patricia Beam and she could comment on my form more often than once a year at the Illinois Senior Olympics.) Before that time no one who knew anything about racewalking had ever seen me racewalk, and I hadn't read anything about the proper form. It's important to carry your head level and keep your chin off your chest to maximize your intake of oxygen. Even with your head up, you can scan down with your eyes to ensure you see rough patches in your path that could cause you to trip.

Jeff Salvage told me this is a common problem with racewalkers, and he attributes it to a lack of focus. No doubt he's right – when I'm walking alone I often catch myself daydreaming, and when I do my head is always down.

The second habit that I picked up on a treadmill is striding too far forward with the lead leg. I lengthened my stride in front as I turned up the speed. Taking a long stride in front with a straightened leg tends to have a braking effect on your forward motion because your body must vault up and over the straightened leg. Walking on a treadmill lessens the braking effect because the treadmill exerts a force toward you that helps your body vault up and over the straightened leg. Thus you don't get penalized by the inefficiency of over-striding with the lead leg when walking on a treadmill as much as you do when walking on a track or roadway.

Finally, I don't think I felt a need to push off with my back foot because the treadmill surface was actively moving away from my foot. My foot just naturally went back, my heel rose up off the surface and I was eventually up on my toes without any force on my own part to extend my ankle or to push off with my toes. I was missing out on that component of racewalking propulsion.

You are better off learning to racewalk on stationary ground, and once you have a feel for the technique you can spend some time training on a treadmill when necessary. If you must learn on a treadmill, you need to understand the basics of technique to avoid the bad habits I picked up.

I received a tip on training on a treadmill in a conversation with a racewalker at the 2007 National Senior Games in Louisville. A couple of years ago he and his racewalking wife purchased a surveillance kit from Radio Shack for about $150. It included two cameras and a monitor. They mounted one camera so that it pointed at knee level from the side and the other at foot level from the front. They put the monitor where they could see it in front of the treadmill, and the picture automatically toggled back and forth from the knee view to the foot view. The arrangement gave instantaneous feedback on straightened knee/toe up form even when no one was around to observe. If they saw something that needed improvement, they could correct it while still walking. I think it's a great idea. You can place the cameras to observe your whole body or zero in on any part of your technique that needs work. Unlike looking at videotape, you see your form as you walk and can reprogram your neuromuscular system to proper technique immediately.

If you own a video camera, you may be able to get real-time feedback while walking on a treadmill. Most cameras allow you to connect your camera to a television or monitor. You can turn on the camera without pushing the "record" button and view images in real time on the television. Place the camera to show the view you want to monitor and watch your form in real time. I ordered a 25-foot video cable on Amazon for less than $6 and can see a live side view of my entire body while walking on the treadmill.

## Parks, Streets and Sidewalks

If you are a runner or a recreational walker, you run or walk somewhere. Maybe you go to a nearby park with a paved path like I do. Perhaps you run or walk on some side streets or empty sidewalks. If these locations work for those activities, they'll generally work for racewalking, too. Two exceptions are steep downhill grades and uneven rocky paths. Salvage warns in *Racewalk Like a Champion* that you should not try to racewalk down a hill if it is so steep that you cannot maintain proper form. Instead walk or jog down the hill. He points out that judged racewalks should not contain hills of that grade.

Paths, streets and sidewalks often have a slope to shed water to the side. If there is a level "crown" where it is safe to walk, I use that. If the crown is in the middle of a roadway, it's probably not safe to walk the crown. On sloped surfaces I even out the stress on my joints by walking part of the time with the slope to my right and part of the time with the slope to my left. Because I usually walk several laps of the path at the park where I train, I even out the wear on my joints by walking half the laps in one direction and half in the other.

Perhaps you are one of the lucky ones with a school track facility nearby that local residents are allowed to use. That makes a great place to train. But don't always go the same direction around the track as always turning in one direction may put uneven wear on your joints. You may want to do some training off the track for two reasons: First, it's boring just going round and round a track. Second, it probably is good to put in a little bit of work up and down slight grades.

## Alone or with Company

I have good friends who are runners, and they tend to run with other people. Some run with another person who has a similar schedule and pace. Others socialize as they run with a group. I also often see runners out chewing up the miles alone.

In the past I mostly walked by myself because there weren't any local racewalkers to train with me. I am able to get out and walk without being prodded by a commitment to others. However, I enjoy spending time teaching others to racewalk. I appreciate the camaraderie and am grateful to get feedback from them on my own form. We get together as a group weekly in a city park, and new recruits show up on a regular basis.

If you have a racewalking club in your area, you are fortunate. You will be able to get help on your technique from the beginning and can avoid picking up bad habits. The club will have suggestions about places to walk, training sessions to work on stamina and technique and races if you want some competition. Several of the Web sites in the Appendix have links to racewalking clubs around the country.

Some road running clubs have racewalking groups within the membership. If you don't have a local racewalking club, check with your local runners' group to see if it includes racewalkers.

Charities often sponsor walks as fundraising events. You can walk in one of these and contribute to a good cause as well as to your good health. Maybe you'll attract some new converts to racewalk too.

If you don't have any fellow racewalkers, go by yourself. I do it for more than two years, and most days I still train alone. I usually encounter the same people running or walking in the park so it's not actually lonely.

If you really don't want to go by yourself, suggest this book to a friend. Train together, observe one another's technique and get off on the right foot.

# Racewalker Profile

**Patricia Beam**
Caledonia, IL
Year of Birth: 1937

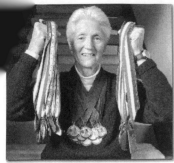

*Photo taken by Sara Garcia*

Patricia Beam, a multi-sport athlete who regularly wins a dozen or more gold medals at the Illinois Senior Olympics, took up racewalking in 1996 when others encouraged her to try it at a senior games. "I did the 1,500 (meter) and the 5,000 (meter) the same morning," she said. "The next day I had very achy legs."

Beam gets most of her racewalk training while walking her neighbor's dog on a 1.5 mile loop. Her racewalking also benefits from her training for bicycle racing, where she competes in time trials, closed short-course criterium races and road races.

"Racewalking is invigorating," claimed Beam. "It provides a wonderful appetite, and you can eat as much of the right food as you desire. After a great racewalk your body knows that it wants only healthy food and beverages." Beam has not had any racewalking injuries.

Beam recommended that someone new to the sport "invest in a good pair of shoes. Watch a race and ask for pointers or get a good video and book," she added.

# Racewalker Profile

**Robert Shires, M.D.**
Des Moines, IA
Year of Birth: 1950

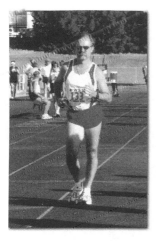

Dr. Robert Shires was a track athlete in high school but got away from running during the rigors of college and medical school. He eventually got back to running but, like so many others, he became injured. "In 1992 I was tired of plantar faciitis and backaches from running so I looked to another aerobic activity," he said. "I investigated racewalking and purchased Martin Rudow's *Advanced Racewalking*. This directed me the American Racewalking Association, which I think has long since dissolved. The association sent me a tape, jacket and reading information. Unlike many of the runners turned-walkers with a good mentor, I was self-taught with the videotape and further reading."

In the mid-1990s Shires attended two clinics by Veisha Sedlak where he picked up tips to help his performance. "A local masters champion, Franklin Brown, encouraged me to continue and improve," Shires added.

When he turned 50, Shires entered the Iowa Senior Olympics and qualified for the 2001 National Senior Games. He won bronze medals in the 1500 meter and 5K races at the nationals. Determined to do even better, Shires increased his training intensity. He won both gold medals in his age group the next three National Senior Games.

Shires alternates between a treadmill and a stationary bicycle during the cold months and trains outdoors during the warm months. He racewalks a hilly, five-mile, residential course three times a week and does speed work on a track on weekends. He works with a trainer one hour a week to maintain leg strength and flexibility.

"My 'healthy pleasure' has given me more energy, better sleep, ─t my weight at ideal for my height and allowed me to compete ─ainst other athletes, which I think keeps me sharper at my profession ─f family medicine," Shires said. "Rarely do I accept excuses from patients that they don't have time to exercise – if I can make time in my hectic schedule so can they."

Shires' only injuries from racewalking have been a couple of days of plantar faciitis after the Las Vegas Half-Marathon in 1999 and the Des Moines Half-Marathon in 2004.

He recommends that newcomers "be patient as it may take up to five months for your hips to stay loose and not create discomfort when racewalking. Veisha always said 'Loose is Power' when racewalking, that is you expend extra energy if you tighten up, especially in the upper body."

# Chapter Six: How Can You Improve?

When I think of improving my racewalking, I consider three things: using better technique, going longer distances and walking faster. The first priority is technique. Take your time getting used to the thrust of your hip pivot forward and the movement of your lead leg up to the heel strike. Work on having your knee straightened at the time of heel strike, keeping your ankle flexed and toe of your shoe up as you rock forward onto the sole of your foot and pushing off as your foot leaves the ground behind you.

When you begin, you probably won't be able to go very far using good technique. The muscles on the front of your legs will not be strong enough to repeatedly hold your ankle flexed and toe up from the time of heel strike until your leg passes under your body. You may not be able to hold your ankle flexed for any duration, and your foot may slap down against the ground soon after your heel contacts the ground. You may be able to keep it flexed for the first few minutes of walking and then the muscle on the front of your leg will tire and give you a burning sensation from the buildup of lactic acid.

This muscle strengthens fairly quickly. Practicing racewalking builds up the muscle, but you also can do some exercises to help strengthen it.

Sometimes I'll sit or stand and just flex my ankles and point my toes upward as high as I can and hold them there for about 30 seconds. Try it. Hold onto something for balance if you do this while standing. You'll probably feel some burning in the muscle after 15 or seconds. Do two or three repetitions of this a few times a day and you'll see progress.

You can improvise weight-lifting exercises. When I'm watching TV, I put my toes under the legs of one end of our coffee table and flex my ankles and toes up to lift the end of the table off the floor. I'll hold it up for a few seconds, slowly let it down and repeat until my shin muscles are exhausted.

Another exercise I use is to take 25 or 30 little steps walking on my heels with my ankle flexed and toes pointed up. Sometimes I sit in a chair with my leg extended and move my ankle in a way that my toes trace out numbers or the alphabet in the air.

Don't forget the earlier guidance about using shoes with low heels. You'll find it much easier to keep your ankle flexed and toe of your shoe up when the heel strike is with a low-heeled shoe rather than a thick-heeled training shoe. It made a noticeable difference for me.


## Training

Racewalking is no different from most other activities. Whether it's playing the piano or racewalking, if you want to get better, you'll have to spend some time at it. Use some common sense. A neophyte might be able to sit down at the piano and peck away at the keys for a few hours and not be any worse for the wear. But if a new racewalker worked out for a few hours, he or she would be exceedingly sore the next day. So take it easy and work up to longer and faster walks gradually. The object is to acquire a skill that brings you a lifetime of better health, and you have a lifetime to improve on that skill.

I vary my training from day to day for four reasons. First, it keeps me fresh if I change my workout a bit each day. Second, it helps prevent injuries if I do different distances and speeds that place different amounts of stress on my body each day. Third, I try to tailor my workouts to upcoming races. If I have a 1,500 meter race upcoming, I'll do a higher percentage of workouts in the lead-up to the race that are shorter and faster than usual. If there is a 10K on the horizon, I'll do a higher percentage of longer, slower workouts. But I'll still do some of each every week.

The fourth reason I vary my workout is that benefits transcend the type of workout one is doing. When I do speed work, it helps me walk at a faster cadence even in longer races. In his clinic Dave McGovern indicated that long, slow workouts build additional blood-carrying capillaries in muscles that help get oxygen to those muscles in short, fast races.

One of my goals in racewalking is to approximate the standard in the book *Younger Next Year* of 45 minutes of exercise 6 days a week at 60 to 65 percent of maximum heart rate. To do this I need to know my maximum heart rate.

Both Salvage and McGovern take issue with the old rule of thumb for calculating one's maximum heart rate, i.e. subtracting one's age from 220.[10] I'm currently 58, so that rule suggests my maximum heart rate is 162 beats per minute. The indicated training range of 60 to 65 percent of my maximum heart rate is 97 to 105 beats per minute.

When calculating a training heart rate Salvage uses a version of the Karvonen Formula, which takes into consideration one's physical conditioning as indicated by resting heart rate. To use the formula you start with 220 and subtract from that your age and your resting heart rate. Multiply that result by the percentage of the maximum rate you want to use in training and then add your resting heart rate to that product. Assume you are age 60, have a resting heart rate of 55 and want to train at 65 percent of your maximum heart rate. The calculation of the formula is shown on the following page.

---

[10] An interesting article entitled "THE SURPRISING HISTORY OF THE 'HRmax=220-age' EQUATION" may be found at *Journal of Exercise Physiologyonline*, Volume 5 Number 2 May 2002 at http://faculty.css.edu/tboone2/asep/Robergs2.pdf . The authors study 30 variants of the equation and conclude that none are sufficiently accurate, although the best fit to the data was the equation HRmax=205.8-(0.685age).

$$[(220 - 60 - 55) \text{ x } .65] + 55 = 65 \text{ percent of maximum heart rate}$$
$$[105 \text{ X } .65] + 55 = 65 \text{ percent of maximum heart rate}$$
$$68.25 + 55 = 65 \text{ percent of maximum heart rate}$$
$$123.25 = 65 \text{ percent of maximum heart rate}$$

In order to use this formula, you must know your resting heart rate. Take your heart rate in the morning while still lying in bed. This is the heart rate to use in the formula.

McGovern calculates an estimated maximum heart rate for participants in his clinics based on results of three increasingly strenuous interval walks with intervening two-minute rest periods. He estimated my maximum heart rate at 180 beats per minute.

If I use the outdated 220 minus your age methodology, it calculates a 65 percent of maximum heart rate training target for me of 105 beats per minute. McGovern's estimate suggests a 65 percent level at 117 beats per minute, and Salvage's formula puts it at 122. McGovern's and Salvage's methodologies give similar results for me and take into consideration my personal characteristics.

Even using the experts' calculations, I've been training above the 65 percent level at 125 to 150 heart beats per minute. Some of the races I train for are 1,500 meter races that last less than 10 minutes. I do some speed work and may only spend a half hour rather than 45 minutes training on some days. Also, since I'm training for races, I'm pushing myself more than one would need to do for good health. You can get great exercise at a slower pace. In fact, in reviewing *Younger Next Year*, I think it might be better for me to move toward longer, slower workouts to get the maximum health benefits Crowley and Lodge envision. I have two goals: good health and competing successfully. My training regimen is a compromise between the two and may not maximize accomplishment of either goal.

I hope to enter some longer races in the future, and if I do, my daily training time will need to expand. I'll also need some expert

guidance for that training. I'd advise you to get some additional adv.
on racewalk training, too.

That expert, detailed guidance on racewalk training can be
found in books and on Web sites by Jeff Salvage and Dave McGovern.
Salvage's book is *Racewalk Like a Champion* and his Web site is
http://www.racewalk.com. McGovern's book is *The Complete Guide
to Racewalking Technique and Training* and his Web site may be
found at www.racewalking.org. They provide guidance on increasing
distance and speed and provide detailed training schedules. I don't
know if I'll ever need McGovern's other book, *The Complete Guide to
Marathon Walking*, but you might.

## Stretching

I don't enjoy stretching even though I know it is good for me.
Some people must like it – I think they're the ones who get into yoga,
which is something I've tried a few times but have trouble continuing.
When McGovern demonstrated stretched at his clinic he remarked that
he doesn't like stretching. Still, he emphasized that it's important.

You should consult other resources about stretching, including
the books and Web sites mentioned previously. You already may have
a stretching routine that you can adapt to your needs as a racewalker. I
remind you, however, to stretch after you have warmed up your
muscles and tendons, not before. The stretching is more effective then,
and you are less likely to injure yourself.

Choose stretches that address the areas of the body that need
flexibility when racewalking: shoulders, waist, hip sockets, fronts and
backs of the legs, ankles and toes. If you feel tightness in a certain
area, that usually indicates you need to work on that location.

When I was at the unexpected clinic in Florida, Frank Alongi
recommended two stretching exercises to me. He noticed that I was
not very flexible, which caused two problems with my form. First, I

1 trouble getting my ankle flexed and toe up to assist in raightening my knee. Second, my hips weren't pivoting sufficiently.

Alongi thought the hamstring muscles located on the back of my thighs were too tight to allow my legs to completely straighten and get my ankles flexed with my toes up. He suggested a stretching exercise in which I stood close to the back of a park bench (the edge of a picnic table or other sturdy furniture would work) and grabbed hold of the back of the bench with both hands. He had me flex my right ankle upward and point the toe of my shoe up as high as I could. Next he had me step back with my left foot as far as possible so that I was on the toes of my left foot with my left heel off the ground. Then he told me to try to push my left heel toward the ground while still trying to hold the toe of my right shoe pointed upward. This put an incredible stretch on the hamstring in the back of my right leg. He had me do this for 30 seconds and then switch legs.

Sometimes I stop during a training session and do this stretch. In addition, I always do it at the end of my workout. I believe it has helped me straighten my leg at the knee, get my ankle flexed with the toe up and avoid red cards in competition.

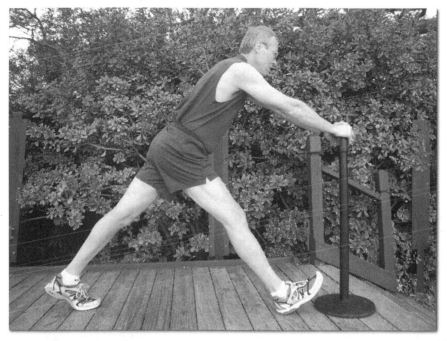

*Figure 6-1: This is the stretch Frank Alongi suggested for stretching my hamstring so it would be easier to flex my ankle and toe upward to get my knee straightened. Flex the ankle of the lead foot upward as far as possible, and then try to push the heel of the trailing foot toward the ground. You'll feel a stretch down the back of the front leg.*

The other exercise Alongi showed me helps loosen the hip pivot. He had me grab hold of the back of the park bench (a post or a wall would work as well) and then step back with both feet so that my body was at about a 45 degree angle with the ground. My body was straight from my head and neck down through my waist and knees. I was up on my toes and my heels were off the ground. He then had me bend my right knee toward the ground and simultaneously pivot my right hip toward the ground. Next, he had me bring the right knee and hip back and bend the left knee and hip toward the ground. He had me repeat this as fast as I could and said I should repeat the cycle 100 or 150 times per day.

I haven't been as faithful with this exercise, and I believe my form and speed have suffered.

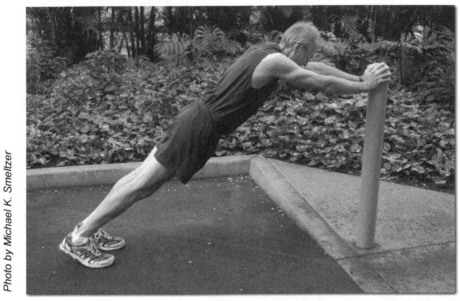

*Figure 6-2: The hip-loosening exercise Frank Alongi recommended started with leaning against a bench, wall or pole with the body and legs straight.*

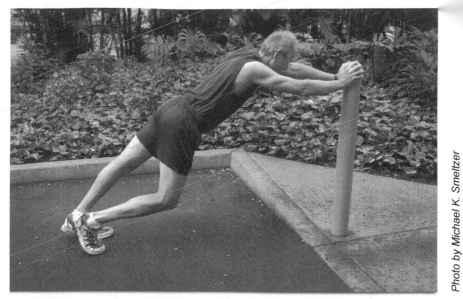

*Figure 6-3: The right knee and the right hip are flexed downward ...*

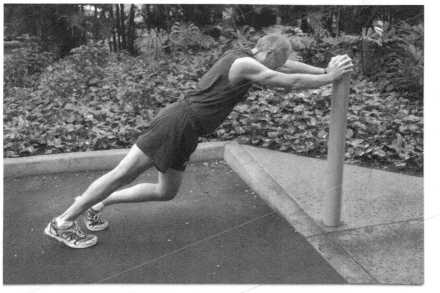

*Figure 6-4: ...and then the right knee and right hip are returned to the starting position as the left knee and left hip are flexed downward. Alongi said to repeat these movements as fast as possible 100 to 150 times.*

As with training and stretching tips, I suggest you consult the aforementioned books and Web sites for various drills to speed up your foot cadence and to add flexibility. One of the drills I do that McGovern used in his clinic and Salvage recommends in his book is a "quick steps" drill in which you racewalk as fast as you can while taking very little steps. You quickly move each foot barely in front of the other. I can't do this for very long, but it seems to speed up my cadence when I go back to regular racewalking.

I do another speedwork drill in which I racewalk as fast as I can for a minute while counting my footsteps. It is difficult to count every heel strike when you are walking quickly so you'll find it easier to count every heel strike by your right foot or your left foot for one minute and then double the number to get your total number of steps. I count my right foot heel strikes for a minute during some drills and in other drills count my left foot heel strikes. I think I subconsciously strike my heel harder on the foot I'm counting, and I want to even out the stress on my legs.

Top racewalkers take 220 or more strides per minute for miles at a time. I can get to 180 strides for 1 minute. Speed drills may help me improve a bit above 180 strides for 1 minute, but it's more likely they will help me keep up a slightly slower cadence for longer periods of time. Sometimes when I'm walking and it feels like I'm loafing and my heart rate isn't up as much as I'd like, I count my footsteps for a minute. It seems that I subconsciously pick up my cadence just because I'm paying attention. It's a trick that I use to keep me focused on days when I feel I'm slacking off.

The drill that improved my technique the most in the shortest time is the "four-minute mirror drill" Bonnie Stein taught me. Kinnan Johnston, who was one of Stein's trainees and now assists her coaching others, had a persistent problem with her arm motion. One session Stein noticed that Johnston's arm movement was much

78

improved. Johnston credited a drill she herself had developed. Bonnie dubbed Johnston's drill the "four-minute mirror drill."

This simple drill consists of standing, facing a mirror and moving your arms in the correct racewalking motion for one minute. Then you turn so your right side is to the mirror and continue for another minute. Next you turn so your left side is to the mirror for a minute. Finally, you again face the mirror for a minute. Your feet don't move.

By watching yourself in the mirror, you can monitor your arm motion in real time and make instantaneous corrections. This is working wonders for me because it enables me to address three major flaws in my form: raising my shoulders, dropping my head and flailing my arms to the side.

You can do this drill every morning when you get up whether you have a chance to get out and racewalk or not. Repetition of proper technique is the key to success. Stein, who has a master's degree in education, said it takes 20,000 repetitions for the neuromuscular system to master a movement.

## Strength Training

Before I began racewalking my strength training involved working out with free weights or machines at a level that exhausted my muscles in 8 to 12 repetitions. I was trying to bulk up my muscles a bit. Since then I've changed my philosophy. I'm now going with lighter weights and more repetitions to build endurance and general strength rather than bulky muscles. Because I'm an ectomorph, the bulking up effort wasn't doing much for me, anyway.

I try to work with weights a couple of times a week although I find it difficult to do that in the summer when the weather's nice and I'm training outdoors. I have to be careful with leg machines. If I do a bit too much, my knees become sore. It's been an enlightening experience. If I lift a moderate amount of weight on a weight machine my knees bother me. However, I can compete in a 10K racewalk and the next morning have no pain. Unlike my basketball playing days, I don't have to ice my knees after racewalking.

Strength training is good for one's general muscle, skeletal and joint health. Crowley and Lodge recommend it in *Younger Next Year*. Salvage and McGovern recommend it in their racewalking books and have some tips on the specific exercises helpful to racewalkers. McGovern also indicates certain work with heavier weights for "explosive" strength may be in order to add speed to one's racewalking.

If you aren't currently doing any strength training, ease into it. Get some guidance from a trainer if you can, but let the trainer know your interest is in endurance and general strength rather than building bulging biceps.

## Practice, Practice, Practice

I ended the chapter on technique with the thought that the way to get the racewalking technique hardwired into your neuromuscular system is to practice, practice and practice. The same is true with improving your speed and lengthening the distance you can racewalk. If you spend time training, stretching and doing drills, you will be rewarded with faster times and more stamina for increased distances.

## Other Resources

I've given you enough knowledge and encouragement to get you off to a great start, but eventually you will want to tap the wisdom of others to assist your progress in the sport. The Appendix contains a list of Web sites that connect you to a wide array of racewalking resources. The sites provide in-depth guidance on technique and training, and they will help you locate books by experts such as Jeff Salvage and Dave McGovern, clinics, competitions and local racewalking clubs. You can't find a better place to work on your technique and speed than a racewalking club, where you can get ongoing analysis and support from fellow walkers.

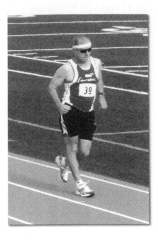

# Racewalker Profile

**Dave Couts**
Whiteside, MO
Year of Birth: 1955

When he was in his late 20s Dave Couts ran a summer youth track club that participated in Junior Olympic meets. Couts convinced some of the kids to enter racewalk events and tried to teach them the technique even though at the time he didn't know all the rules. Over the course of a few meets his athletes figured out what they needed to do to walk legally, and three qualified for the national meet.

A few years later Couts, a 5K and 10K runner, experienced nagging ankle and Achilles' tendon problems and decided to try racewalking as a competitive alternative. Then living near Kansas City, he sought out the Heartland Racewalkers for instruction.

"I remember when I first went there, and they took me out to see what my form looked like," Couts said. "I wanted to go just as fast as I could. My knees were bent. I probably looked like Groucho Marx sprinting in the parking lot. I learned that I needed to slow down to learn the technique. Then I could pick up speed later. People need to realize that racewalking is a discipline with certain criteria that must be met to be legal."

Couts now belongs to the Racewalkers' Club of St. Louis and trains in various parks. "I've learned if I stop and train on the way home (from work) I'll do it," he said, "but if I get home and sit down it's hard to get motivated. I don't have anyone to train with, but (a training partner) would be a good motivator."

He stays active throughout the year playing basketball and softball, and he sometimes runs. He said he's had his share of injuries during the years from various sports, but racewalking injuries have been "mostly hamstring pulls from not warming up enough. Some of mine are age and repetition injuries," he added.

Couts competes frequently and has been successful, including winning both the 1,500 meter and 5K racewalking events in the 50-54 age group at the 2007 National Senior Games. But it isn't only about competition. "It's what I do to relax," he said. "Even if I didn't compete, I love to go out and train."

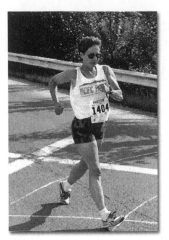

# Racewalker Profile

**Bev McCall**
Mazama, WA
Year of Birth: 1936

Bev McCall was a frequently injured distance and endurance athlete when she discovered racewalking in 1980. A weekly column and event information on racewalking in a Seattle-area running magazine and a couple of knowledgeable racewalkers who gave free weekly instruction helped her get started. The Pacific Pacers Racewalk Club "has been a great source of support, especially in the first few years," McCall said. "Equally important, it's been something I can contribute to in terms of time and expertise."

"I've competed a lot for 25 years," McCall said. In recent years she progressively decreased her training from 50 miles per week to 20 miles per week, but she increases her mileage when getting ready for specific events. McCall generally trains on pavement but occasionally works out on a track. She has had only a few racewalking injuries during her career, and none lasted more than a week.

McCall's health and weight have been stable for years, and she said training and competition also are good for mental health.

"Connect to a club or other walkers," McCall said. "Think about your purpose – be realistic. Make it part of your life for the long haul."

# Chapter Seven: Are You Ready for Some Competition?

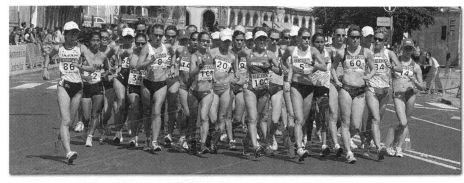

*Photo by Jeff Salvage*

*Figure 7-1: 2006 20K Women's World Cup*

The prospect of athletic competition initially attracted me to racewalking. It's a sport for which I could train vigorously without injury and in which I felt I could have some competitive success. Anticipation of upcoming competitions gave me an incentive to work on my conditioning and technique.

I continue to look forward to competing in races, and I try to adjust my training in light of the specific distance of an upcoming race. If my next race is a 1,500 meter event, I'll do some extra speed work. If it's a 10K, I'll do some longer walks in preparation.

I would continue to racewalk even if I had no future competitions. I enjoy the activity itself and appreciate the benefits to my cardiovascular, muscular and skeletal systems. At this point, however, I want to continue to compete. Perhaps you want some competition, too. I can help you find it.

## Finding Events for Competition

My first racewalk competition was in the Illinois Senior Olympics. Almost every state offers a senior games competition, and they all use the same five-year age groupings – 50-54, 55-59, 60-64, etc. The National Senior Games Association (NSGA) Web site (http://www.nsga.com/about.html) contains a directory of state games that indicates the dates they are held and contact information.

The state games generally have their own Web sites that may be accessed from the NSGA site. The state sites identify the events offered at the games. Most states offer a 1,500 meter racewalk event or a 5K racewalk event, and some have both. Many sites also provide recent results. You can check the times to see how your training times match up with the competition. You may find there were fewer contestants in your age group than awards offered so anyone who completed the race without being disqualified got a medal.

You also may find events at the state games that interest you in addition to the racewalk. In my first competition I also long jumped and high jumped. In another I shot basketball free throws and cast fishing plugs for accuracy.

Most states do not require one to qualify at a local senior games in order to compete in the state games. Check your state games rules to be certain. Also, most states have "open" games, i.e. out-of-state competitors are welcome to participate. This offers additional opportunities for competition. The two impressive racewalkers in my first Illinois Senior Olympics experience were from Missouri and Iowa.

The National Senior Games are held in the summer of odd-numbered years. Participants must qualify at a state senior games in the calendar year preceding the national games. For example, athletes must have qualified at a state senior games in 2008 to be eligible for the 2009 National Senior Games in San Francisco and must qualify in 2010 to be eligible for the 2011 National Senior Games in Houston.

You must place first, second or third in your age and gender group in a state racewalk competition to qualify for the national games. In some years qualification may be extended to fourth-place finishers. If you happen to be in a state with a large number of especially good athletes, additional competitors may qualify if their times meet certain age-group standards set by the National Senior Games Association. Also, it doesn't matter if your state only offers one racewalk distance. If you qualify at the state level for either the 1,500 meter or 5K racewalk, you may enter both races at the National Senior Games.

The state games that allow out-of-state competitors provide additional opportunities to qualify for the national games. In 2008 I qualified for the 2009 National Senior Games through summer competitions in Iowa and Missouri before the Illinois Senior Olympics were held in September. Qualifying in another state may act as a safety net for the national games if you happen to be injured or ill when your own state's qualifying games are scheduled.

If your state allows out-of-state competitors, it does not hurt your chances of qualifying for the National Senior Games. An out-of-state racewalker who places in the top three in a given age group qualifies for the national games, but the first three in-state competitors in that age group also qualify.

Many states also have local games. Some, as in Florida, may be affiliated with the state senior games, but others are independent. A state's official state senior games' Web site may list local senior games. A phone call or email to the state games authorities may generate a list of local games. Entering something like the words "senior Olympics games Illinois" (without the quotation marks) into an Internet search engine such as Google will likely turn up local games if they exist. The Huntsman World Senior Games (www.seniorgames.net), which are held each fall in St. George, Utah, include racewalking events of several distances.

Racewalking clubs often sponsor races for their members and others. Several of the Web sites listed in the Appendix have links to racewalking clubs by state along with Web addresses or contact information for the clubs. Dave McGovern's Web site (www.racewalking.org) has an extensive calendar of upcoming racewalks. *WALK! Magazine's* Web site (www.walk-magazine.com/index.html) has a calendar of walks although many may not be competitions in which racewalking technique is judged.

USA Track & Field (USATF), the official governing body for track and field, long-distance running and racewalking in the United States, oversees annual racewalking national championship competitions of distances from 1 mile to 50 kilometers. In some years USATF includes a 100 kilometer championship. Check the USATF Web site (www.usatf.org/) for information about the races. Participants must be members of USATF, and only United States citizens are eligible for championship awards. For most championship races you don't need to meet performance standards to participate so the not-so-good are free to compete with the best. In some competitions, USATF recognizes awards in five-year increments for masters athletes age 40 and older. The USATF Web site also includes an Events/Calendar section with a search feature you can use to find upcoming racewalking events across the country.

On the www.masterstrack.com Web site you can find masters track meets by state. You generally can use links from the site to find if a racewalk is one of the events in the track meet. This Web site and the USATF Web site both contain the same national masters racewalking rankings for men and women by five-year age groups for various distances for each calendar year. Someone culls this information from the results of various races. A further link to the masters racewalking races that were used in compiling that list is helpful. For 2006 there were 218 separate masters racewalking races used to generate the rankings list. You can use this list to see the

88

names, locations and dates of races that have been held in past years. This, along with Internet search engines and other tools, should help you locate the date and location of the same race in future years.

World Masters Athletics (www.world-masters-athletics.org), formerly World Association of Veteran Athletes, sponsors an Olympics-style track and field competition in odd-numbered years for athletes in age groups beginning with age 35. The 2009 meet is in Lahti, Finland, and the 2011 competition is scheduled for Sacramento, California. The racewalking events include a 5K for men and women, a 10K for women and a 20K for men.

Organizers of some road races advertise them as walker-friendly and even may have an earlier start time for walkers. That's how I did my first 10K race. Walkers got a 30-minute head start. If I were a really good racewalker, none of the fastest runners in the field of nearly 1,000 would have caught me. A few did, but it was fun crossing the finish line walking in the midst of some of the very best runners.

If you are unsure whether walkers are welcome in a local road race, check with the race director before signing up. In most local road races, some people jog slowly or alternate running and walking so a racewalker is unlikely to be the last one to finish.

When I'm racewalking in a road race, I wear one of my shirts that has "racewalk" or "racewalking" on it. (They are available on www.boomerwalk.com as well as on Salvage's and McGovern's Web sites.) I do it partly to inform spectators about racewalking and partly so people won't think I have a really unusual running style. In my first 10K I wore a racewalking singlet made of a fancy, sweat-wicking material that was more chafing than I realized. Afterward an experienced road runner friend found me in the crowd and said, "You've got bloody nipples!" I looked down to see two pink streaks down the front of my shirt. "Guys are supposed to put Band-Aids over their nipples for distance races," she said. So far that's my worst racewalking injury.[11]

## Avoiding Disqualification

After you've gone to the effort of training for a judged race, it would be a bummer to get disqualified. Don't be too discouraged if that happens, however. Some of the best walkers get disqualified now and then. As I said earlier, in my first race at the National Senior Games judges pulled the man in second place off the track as he was coming down the home stretch.

Be sure to wear appropriate clothing. Generally, one must wear shorts that are sufficiently above the knee to give the judges an adequate view of the leg and knee. Recent styles in workout clothes tend to include shorts that end just above the knee, and those are too long. In colder weather, judges may allow tights, but they must be snug to the leg so the judges get a good view of the leg and knee.

Before you go to your first judged competition, it might be a good idea to look through the Racewalking Officials Handbook. It is accessible as a pdf file on the USATF Web site. (Go to http://www.usatf.org/groups/Racewalking/officials/ and then click on "Racewalking Officials Handbook.") The handbook identifies details judges look for and the kinds of behaviors that may attract a judge's attention and cause the judge to focus on a specific racewalker for special scrutiny.

A judge may give a racewalker a warning if it appears the competitor is close to breaking one of the rules. The judge notifies the racewalker of the caution by holding a yellow paddle. One side of the paddle has a ~ symbol on it and indicates the athlete is in danger of having both feet off the ground. The other side has a > symbol that indicates a bent knee infraction is at risk.

---

[11] Robert Shires told me about NipGuards, a product specifically designed to address this problem. You can read the poem Shires wrote about the product following the Las Vegas half marathon in the testimonial section of www.nipguards.com.

If a judge observes an actual infraction, that judge will record a red card for the racewalker. If a competitor receives red cards from three different judges, he or she will be disqualified from the race. It is important to note that a racewalking judge can only issue each athlete a red card once per race. In some races officials place a disqualification posting board in sight of the contestants so that each can see if he or she has accumulated any red cards during the race. The offending racewalker is put on notice of the offense and perhaps can correct the technique before being issued a second or third red card. In races where a posting board is not available, the chief judge is responsible for notifying competitors of accumulated red cards during the race. In a short race the judge might not have time for notification, and you could learn of disqualification after the race.

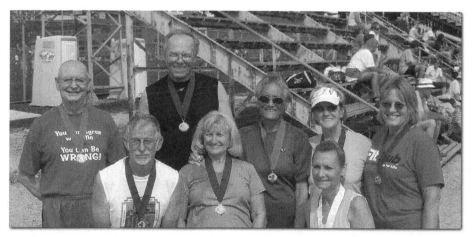

*Figure 7-2: Several racewalkers trained by the author entered the 2008 Illinois Senior Olympics 1500 meter racewalk event. None were disqualified for rule infractions, all won age-group medals and each qualified for the National Senior Games in 2009. Front row, from left to right: Duane Wilson, Joyce Ludwig and Lois Stone. Back row: Bill Thomas, Brent Bohlen, Kate Kanaley Miller, Jan Wilson and Marilyn Cisco. (Photo by Chuck Ludwig)*

# Racewalker Profile

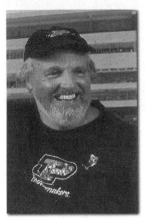

**John McGinty**
Indianapolis, IN
Year of Birth: 1937

One day in 1989 after his usual jogging regimen, John McGinty felt especially good and ran some 400 meter sprints that were not part of his normal training. The next day he realized he had severely damaged his knees.

"After about a year of recovery, I got back on the track and started walking, each time a little faster," he said. "Before long I entered a 5K race as a walker. My intention was to walk a few races before running another one. Watching others do the correct technique and (being) amazed at their speed, I discovered that racewalking was a real sport and not just a courtesy for those who can't run."

McGinty joined the Indiana Racewalkers' Club for a while and now is a member of the Kokomo Roadrunners. The club has a number of racewalkers and offers a racewalk division in most of its road races.

He has competed in senior Olympics since 1993 and has participated in states from California to Florida. He does not limit himself to racewalking but competes in many events including tennis, table tennis, badminton, basketball, swimming and running. He won four national awards in shuffleboard and once competed in 24 events in one day.

McGinty walks two or three miles every other day when training for a race. His only injuries from racewalking were pulled muscles. "In contrast," he said, "I've had more injuries in running than I ever had in football and basketball." The benefits he found from racewalking include increased energy, a low resting heart rate (50 BPM), greater stamina and association with "healthy, friendly, intelligent athletes."

"Athletes new to racewalking would do well to learn the correct technique from an instructor," McGinty advised. "There is a fluidity of motion that novices need to master if they want to take up this sport seriously. The rewards are great, and the races are especially fun. For those who persist the benefits are many."

# Racewalker Profile

**Kate Marrs**
Milwaukee, WI
Year of Birth: 1928

Kate Marrs has the right attitude about age. "I began racewalking 10 years ago when I was just 69," she said.

She was jogging to keep in shape, but her children were concerned she would "wreck" her knees. A daughter sent her an article about racewalking. "I was very much interested but rapidly realized I would never learn it alone. So I went online and found the Parkside Athletic Club. One reason I have continued to work and train is this great group."

Marrs generally trains outdoors and follows a schedule provided by her coach. When the weather is bad, she uses an indoor facility. She said she once overextended herself at a competition and suffered from dehydration.

"I had never competed in anything except a women's tennis league until I began racewalking," Marrs said. "My proudest moment was achieving a world (age-group) record in the indoor 3K at Boston in 2004 – the year after I turned 75."

Marrs believes the older you get the more persistent you have to be about staying in shape. "I notice the difference in how I feel very quickly if I go several days or weeks without working out," she said. It shouldn't all feel like work, though. "Diligence is fine and necessary, but it should still be pleasurable."

# Epilogue: What Is in Our Future?

I'll be racewalking as far into the future as I can see. This past summer I entered several races in nearby states. One of the competitors in four of the races was Tom Young, age 91. Young was encouraged to take up racewalking by his neighbor and fellow Kansas nonagenarian, Jean Brunnenkant, who is profiled after Chapter One. On an extremely hot and muggy June morning in Des Moines, Young racewalked both the 1,500 meter and 5K events. I can't see as far into the future as age 91, but with the example of athletes such as Tom Young, I'll keep looking.

The local road runners club trains a group of about 400 new runners and fitness walkers each summer in preparation for a 10K race. Last year the club let me train about 20 racewalkers for the event. The racewalkers ranged in age from mid-20s to early 70s. On our third night of practice the technique just "clicked" with one of the trainees. Her form was better than mine after two and a half years of practice. For others it has come more slowly, but we all are getting better.

I expect the road runners club will allow racewalkers to be part of the training again and anticipate some of last year's trainees will become this year's trainers. We should have many more racewalkers. I'm no longer the only racewalker in town.

I'd like racewalking to be a part of your future, too. It's good for you. It's great aerobic exercise. It's low impact. It can be social or solitary, whichever you prefer. With a bit of dedication and luck, you can racewalk into your 90s.

I hope tens of thousands of baby boomers join you in taking up the sport. If a critical mass takes up the sport, then corporations will take note, and we'll get a better selection of racewalking shoes.

But mainly it would be a satisfying legacy to know that many people discovered the health benefits of racewalking through this book. I want those of my generation to enjoy a sport that is fun and healthy and can keep us going well into old age. We should be less of a burden on Medicare, but I think we'll draw Social Security longer.

Although it's against my best interest, I'd like to see many of you become racewalking competitors, too. I'm sure lots of you will be much faster walkers than I. If this book convinces you to take up racewalking, I'll be satisfied if you let me know that as you pass me in a race. I'll be the tall guy looking at his feet.

# Appendix – Online Resources

The Web sites below offer a tremendous amount of information about racewalking, but the list is not exhaustive. Many of the Web sites below have links to other relevant sites, and you can discover additional sites using your favorite search engine. Web addresses sometimes change. If an address doesn't work, try putting the site name in a search engine to locate a new address.

http://www.boomerwalk.com

This site introduces the BoomerWalk idea. Learn why baby boomers should be racewalking. Video clips of excellent racewalkers show you how the pieces of racewalking technique fit together fluidly in a sport that is aerobic, low impact and, for some, competitive.

http://www.philsport.com/narf/

One of the best parts of the North American Racewalking Foundation's site is Racewalking 101, a tutorial on racewalking that uses an animated stick figure to demonstrate the various aspects of racewalking technique. The site also includes information on the history of racewalking and other aspects of the sport. The online store includes books and videos about racewalking, and the site has links to racewalking clubs around the country.

http://www.racewalk.com

Jeff Salvage's site has excellent sections on technique and training as well as links to other resources including racewalking clubs around the country. You can buy Salvage's book, *Racewalk Like a Champion*, and the companion video or DVD on the site.

http://www.racewalking.org

Dave McGovern's site includes many articles about racewalking, a schedule of Dave's racewalking clinics and camps, schedules and results of racewalks, training schedules and links to racewalking clubs around the country. You can buy racewalking apparel and many racewalking videos and books at the site, including McGovern's *The Complete Guide to Racewalking Technique and Training* and *The Complete Guide to Marathon Walking*.

http://www.acewalker.com/

Bonnie Stein's site contains dozens of articles on racewalking divided into sections on topics such as Training/Technique, Nutrition and Weight Loss, Motivation, Racewalking in Judged Races and Injury Prevention. She also offers lessons and seminars.

http://www.usatf.org/

This is the official site for USA Track & Field, "the National Governing Body for track and field, long-distance running and racewalking in the United States." The site includes an Events/Calendar section with a search feature that can be used to find upcoming racewalking events.

The "Resources for ..." drop down menu has a "Masters Athletes" section that contains age-group records for track and field events including racewalking and annual age-group rankings of track and field events including racewalking. The rankings are divided by year, gender, age group and distance. The racewalker section also has a link that identifies all of the races that were considered in developing the rankings that can be used to help find future races. Under "Sports" on the Web site a drop-down menu with a "Racewalking" option takes you to a section with additional information about racewalking. Of

98

particular note in the racewalking section, if you click on "Officials" and then click on "Racewalking Officials Handbook," you will get to a 69-page pdf document that explains how racewalks are judged and what judges look for in determining whether a racewalker is walking within the rules.

http://www.masterstrack.com/

The Masters Track site includes links to masters and all-comers track meets by state and includes results from those meets. Some of those track meets have racewalk events. The site also contains the age-group records for track and field events including racewalking and annual age-group rankings of track and field events including racewalking similar to the USATF Web site.

http://www.walk-magazine.com/

The "WALK! Magazine" site has some helpful links to clubs and events. You can read a sample copy of the magazine online for free.

http://www.nsga.com/

The National Senior Games Association site provides information on the biennial National Senior Games (the International Olympic Committee will not let them use the term "Olympics," although most states do) and provides links to annual state senior Olympics. There are dozens of sporting events in addition to the racewalk, and many athletes participate in multiple events. Most states allow out-of-state participants. Many senior athletes participate in several states around the country each year. Most states have 1,500 meter and/or 5K racewalk events.

http://www.seniorgames.net

The Huntsman World Senior Games held each fall in St. George, Utah, include several racewalking distances.

http://www.youngernextyear.com/

The book *Younger Next Year* by Chris Crowley and Henry S. Lodge, M.D., convinced me that I needed to find an aerobic exercise activity that I could do 45 minutes a day for the rest of my life. This official site contains blogs, journals, forums, articles and success stories. There also are links to ordering the author's books if you can't find them at your local bookstore.

# About the Author

Brent Bohlen has been a prosecutor, a budget analyst, a utilities regulator and legal counsel for a taxpayer organization. But most of all he has been an athlete. From the time in the third grade when he joined the junior high track team until his knees forced him to give up basketball for the final time in his early 50s, he participated in organized sports. He thought his competitive days were over until he discovered racewalking, an activity that was kind to his body but as challenging as any sport he had done previously.

Bohlen felt compelled to share his racewalking experience with his fellow baby boomers. *BoomerWalk* is the result.

The author's interests include writing, traveling, fishing and gardening. For 17 years he owned and operated an orchard that produced more than 50 varieties of antique and modern apples, many of which were picked from trees he grafted.

Bohlen's family includes his wife, Mary, who is a university professor and department chair. Their son, Will, is communications director for an international non-governmental organization, and their daughter, Elizabeth, is a kindergarten teacher.